Plague, Pox & Pestilence

PLAGUE, POX & PESTILENCE

Edited by Kenneth F. Kiple

Weidenfeld & Nicolson
London

First published in Great Britain 1997
by Weidenfeld & Nicolson

Text, design and layout copyright © George Weidenfeld & Nicolson, 1997

The acknowledgments on p.176 constitute an extension to this copyright page

A CIP catalogue record for this book is available from the British Library
ISBN 0 297 82254 3

Picture researcher: Elaine Willis
Designed by: The Design Revolution
Typeset in: Garamond 3

Weidenfeld & Nicolson
The Orion Publishing Group
5 Upper St Martin's Lane
London WC2H 9EA

CONTENTS

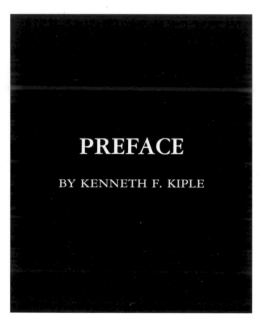

PREFACE

BY KENNETH F. KIPLE

Disease is not a human invention. Rather it is a biological process as old as life itself. Yet, in the pages that follow, we will try to make it clear that over the course of their short stay on earth humans have helped to create their plagues, poxes and pestilence by unwittingly fashioning the kinds of circumstances that brought them forth and then, at times, almost compulsively improving those circumstances so that the diseases flourished.

The reason for this is that humans, unlike their predecessors at the top of the food chain, have not been content simply to live on (and off of) the planet. For at least the last 40,000 years and especially the last 10,000, they have diligently labored to rearrange it. We call such rearranging 'progress', but not always confidently; at times progress seems a kind of ecological Russian roulette that sooner or later will impose the ultimate penalty on us for undoing nature without knowing what we are doing. One relatively modern example is the acceleration of the process of forests turning into farms and farms becoming urban and industrial sprawl. Such a progression makes us uneasy as we hear of holes in the atmosphere and myriad chemicals in the air while watching the shrinking of the forests themselves, which are, after all, the lungs of the globe. But attention wavers because these are long-term concerns about the kind of world future generations will inherit; and there is always the expectation – for some a conviction – that progress itself will rescue us from this fallout of progress.

For some reason, however, we are even more careless of, or oblivious to, other, immediate results of technological lunges. AIDS, the most recent of our plagues, is first and foremost a consequence of progress – in this case of populations moving into rainforests, crisscrossing them with highways, and, in the process, linking all parts of the globe with a previously isolated and unknown virus. The recent fright occasioned by the incredibly fast-acting and deadly Ebola virus constitutes another such example of progress impelling people in the forests toward new and exotic pathogens.

Moving epidemiologically to the opposite side of the 'forest to urban and industrial sprawl' paradigm, progress has placed those of us in the developed world squarely in the midst of a cancer epidemic. It is said that we brought this on ourselves by living long enough to get the disease (also progress of sorts), and there is doubtless considerable truth in the assertion. Yet, to pluck a single oncological example from the many that present themselves, the incidence of skin cancers is increasing – sometimes skyrocketing – wherever statistics are kept. A major cause of these cancers is the ultraviolet component of sunlight, and we have lately begun gazing at the heavens with the not unreasonable suspicion that changes in ultraviolet intensity are occurring because of atmospheric pollution.

That human progress breeds disease, and has always done so, is the theme of this book whose pages focus on twenty-six examples in five different historical categories. Mostly these are a straightforward matter of ecological changes born of progress that have created favorable environments for macro- and micro-parasites and their vectors. But not always. Nutritional diseases such as scurvy are the products of progress but not of pathogens, and other ailments such as epilepsy might appear to have more to do with genetics than with ecological change. But even here we cannot be certain, especially when we learn that it is a disease of multiple causes, among them lead-based paints and drug addiction – two of the more unpleasant products of progress.

In the final section of the book, entitled 'Ephemeral Infirmity', we are forced to relent somewhat on the plagues of progress theme. After all it seems unfair to blame progress for diseases whose identities and causes remain unknown. On the other hand, given its implication in our first twenty-three pestilential examples, some suspicion seems justified.

Hippocrates and Galen.
Thirteenth-century fresco
in Anagni Cathedral,
Italy.

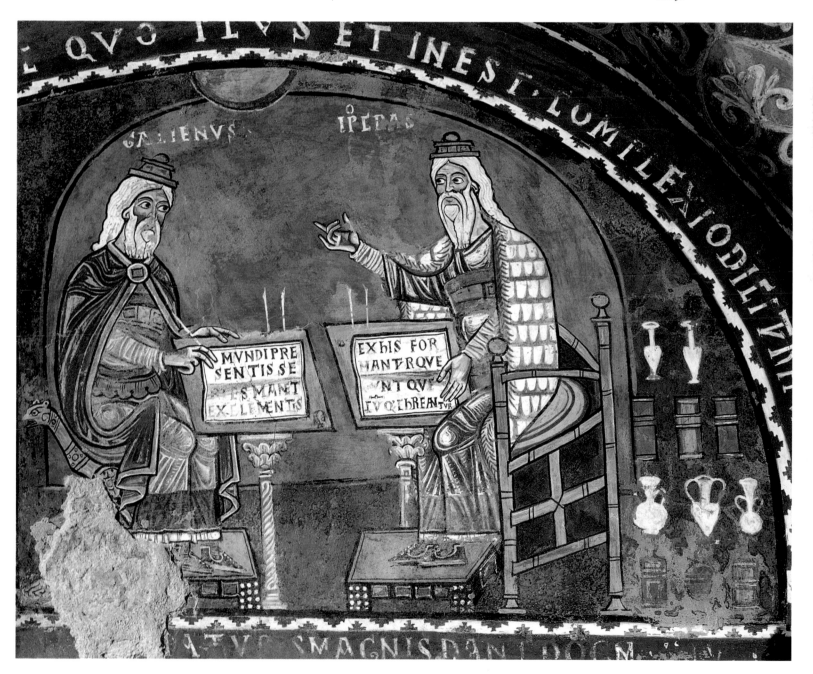

SICKNESS AND SEDENTISM

It was about 40,000 years ago that *Homo sapiens*, the very wise man, appeared on earth. He was the product of an evolutionary journey that had begun with distant primate ancestors – an odyssey that spanned millions of years, during which the various versions of burgeoning humans progressed from making their living as scavengers and gatherers to becoming hunters and gatherers.

As hunter-gatherers they lived in small, isolated bands that moved frequently, which meant few children, because everything had to be carried. It also meant that they seldom remained in one place long enough to pollute water supplies, and let garbage and wastes pile up to attract disease-spreading insects and rodents. In short, small groups that were highly mobile were probably little troubled by disease – especially the contagious illnesses of the microparasites such as measles or influenza, which require large numbers of people to host them. Equally importantly, most of these diseases originally came from those domesticated animals that also provided humans with eggs, milk and meat – and domesticating animals was something that (save for the dog) hunter-gatherers never got around to doing.

The parasites that did make a living off of hunter-gatherers, then, would have been mostly of the macro variety – intestinal worms, lice, fleas and the like, that had adapted to and evolved with humans over the aeons. In addition, humans were doubtless affected from time to time by the parasites of wild animals. The latter are reservoirs for African trypanosomiasis, leptospirosis, relapsing fever, brucellosis, salmonellosis, tularemia, malaria, yellow fever and a host of other ailments. But because a hunter-gathering lifestyle was also prophylactic against vectors shuttling pathogens from person to person, these illnesses would most likely have made isolated appearances but seldom, if ever, affected the whole group.

Moreover, hunter-gatherers ate such a wide range of foods that they could not have developed the deficiency diseases that appeared only as people became more 'civilized'. Interestingly, too, the remains of hunter-gatherers indicate that, at least in terms of protein, their nutritional status was superior to that of almost all who came after them. It is only now that human heights are again approaching those of our ancient ancestors.

Ironically, the good health apparently enjoyed by foragers led ultimately to their becoming farmers. Bands that grew too large to function efficiently subdivided; game animals became scarcer, and humans more numerous; and during the last Ice Age population pressure forced new groups to strike out from the Old World to Australia, Oceania and the Americas until eventually people filled practically every nook and cranny on earth.

In the Americas, the end of the Ice Age and the retreat of the glaciers allowed the pioneers who had crossed the Bering Straits to spread out into a new world full of animal protein for the taking. But in the Old World populations continued to press on one another, animal protein became increasingly scarce, and people who had harvested wild grasses as a seasonal part of their diet began to tinker with them until, finally, they learned to cultivate what would become modernday wheat, rye, barley and rice. The fields attracted wild sheep and goats which were captured and domesticated. Pigs, cattle and fowl followed to fill up barnyards, and by 8,000 or so years ago the Neolithic revolution was well underway.

In the process everything that had protected hunter-gatherers from disease and poor nutrition was turned upside down. The new farmers who now stayed put to concentrate their energies mostly on a single crop needed all the hands they could get for the fields. Birthrates soared even higher than the high infant and child mortality rates, and as village populations swelled, so did their capacity for hosting disease. Humans and their domestic animals living cheek to jowl fouled the water they drank and the soil they walked upon. The squalid conditions of the villages offered a paradise to another set of animals – rats, mice, ticks, flies and mosquitoes – all of which would sooner or later become adept at spreading one or more of the diseases that were now incubating as pathogens ricocheted back and forth between animals and their owners. Human diet deteriorated rapidly as a concentration on tending and consuming a single crop robbed bodies of important nutrients and, consequently, of the ability to resist disease. In short, the Neolithic revolution that we are accustomed to regarding as a giant step upward on the ladder of progress was, in terms of human health, a backward tumble that transformed tall and robust hunter-gatherers into shorter, weaker farmers.

Anemia is the first of three diseases in this section that illustrate something of this physically debilitating ordeal. This illness can be caused by a diet low in iron, such as one based on a lot of one cereal and just a little animal protein, but it can also be triggered by several roundworms, whipworms or hookworms – parasitic boarders that force their hosts to share whatever nutrients the diet provides. Doubtless both instances applied to the first farmers. In the Americas, because the shift from foraging to farming came later than in the Old World, there is much more skeletal evidence of the stresses such a change imposed. And that evidence shows with crystal clarity the absence of anemia in hunter-gatherers and its overwhelming presence in those settled into a life of sedentary agriculture.

Typhoid is a second illness that thrived among sedentary agriculturalists. Probably their first disease encouraging activity was lingering around sources of water long enough to pollute them with human wastes, and because the disease spreads via the oral–fecal route through contaminated food and, especially, water, soon everybody would have been exposed. But not everyone would have become ill.

A distinctive feature of the disease is its existence in a large number of asymptomatic carriers, who would have guaranteed its continual reappearance in local water supplies as well as its spread to other villages, while not succumbing to the disease themselves.

A final example of the diseases the new farmers brought on themselves is schistosomiasis. The first agricultural civilizations appeared in riparian environments – such as the Tigris and Euphrates valley, the Nile and the Yellow River where irrigation farming could be practiced. Irrigation had the beneficial effect of drowning the weeds that would otherwise compete with the crop under cultivation, but the warm and shallow waters of flooded fields were propitious to the development of the blood fluke (*Schistoma*) that uses the aquatic snail as an intermediary host, and penetrates the skin of humans wading in the water whenever the opportunity is presented. The result was one more dependent for the new farmers to support.

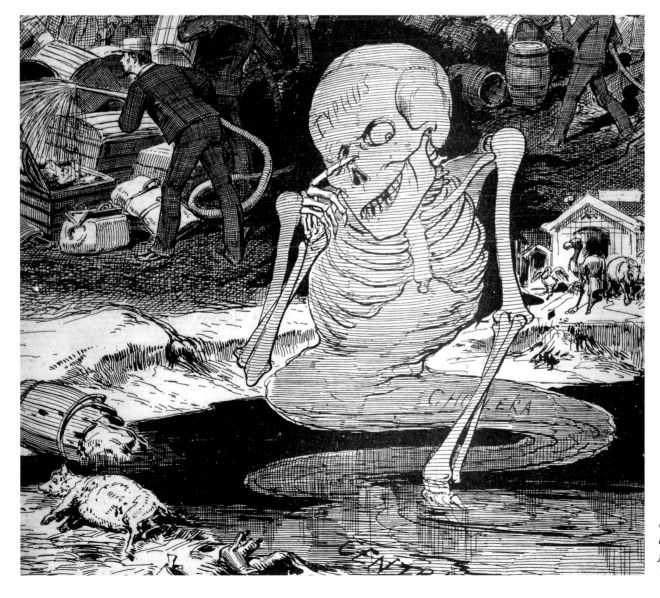

Cartoon warning of contagious miasma arising from Central Park lake. 1885 woodcut, New York.

The study by anthropologists of ancient remains of prehistoric peoples from around the world indicates that anemia has a long history in humans, becoming especially prevalent when people began settling into permanent villages and towns and raising crops. Clearly, this is a disease of sedentism and civilization.

Anemia is present in an individual when either the number of red blood cells or the level of hemoglobin – the chemical on the surface of red blood cells responsible for the transport of oxygen – is below normal. Anemias are either genetic or acquired. Genetic anemias (abnormal hemoglobin), include a range of illnesses, such as sickle cell anemia, found in African and African-diaspora populations, and thalassemia, encountered in Mediterranean groups. Acquired anemias are responses to any nongenetic condition leading to low iron availability. The most common type of acquired anemia is iron deficiency anemia, which has an incidence today of some half-billion in the world's population of 4.5 billion.

Iron was called *sideros* (star) by the ancient Greeks, who believed it to be a gift from the gods. It was used as a therapeutic agent by the ancient Egyptians and Romans, and was recognized by the nineteenth-century French physician, Pierre Blaud as an important treatment for the disease known as the 'green sickness', or 'chlorosis'. Chlorosis was blamed on the sexual excesses of youth, and was depicted by medieval Dutch painters as a disease of young women, with their pale olive complexions a prominent symptom.

Iron bioavailability is influenced by a variety of factors. Dietary sources are determined by the kind of food eaten, either heme or nonheme. Heme iron – meat, fish and poultry are especially good sources – is most easily and efficiently absorbed. Iron found in meat does not require processing in the stomach, and the amino acids from meat digestion help to enhance iron absorption. Nonheme iron is found in plants and is the major source of iron for humans, but is less efficiently absorbed. Moreover, various substances in some plants actually inhibit iron absorption, such as phytates in many nuts (e.g. almonds, walnuts), cereals (e.g. maize, rice, whole wheat flour) and legumes (e.g. peas). By contrast, a number of foods contain substances that serve as iron enhancers, such as ascorbic acid. Citric acid from various fruits and lactic acid from fermented cereal beers also promote iron absorption. Additionally, absorption of nonheme iron in maize is enhanced considerably, by as much as 300 percent, when consumed with fish or meat.

CHAPTER 1

ANEMIA AND THE ANCIENTS

By Clark Spencer Larsen

Advertisement for medicine for the treatment of all manner of illnesses, including the 'green sickness', anemia.

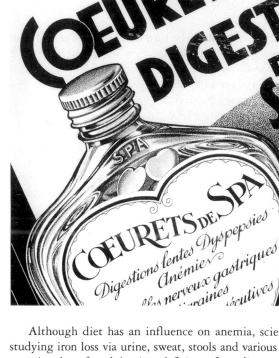

Although diet has an influence on anemia, scientists studying iron loss via urine, sweat, stools and various other secretions have found that iron deficiency from dietary causes is rare. Because most drinking water and natural foods contain appreciable amounts of iron, even the most spartan diets rarely lead to iron deficiency anemia. Indeed, the presence of skeletal evidence of anemia in wild nonhuman primates – who arguably have adequate diets – also suggests that diet by itself is not a leading cause of iron deficiency anemia.

Other more important factors have been identified as contributing to anemia in human populations today. Children with low birth weights are predisposed to anemia. Blood loss, hemorrhage and chronic diarrhea have also been strongly implicated. Parasitic infections can result in blood loss and associated depletion of iron stores. The tropical disease schistosomiasis ('snail fever') triggers an immune response by the body after the eggs of the blood-vessel-inhabiting worms (genus *Schistosoma*) become lodged in organs such as the liver, intestines and urogenital tract. Hookworm disease results from eating or inhaling infective larvae of the hookworm (genera *Ancylostoma duodenale*, *Necator americanus*). The worm literally extracts blood from the human host by grasping the host's intestinal wall with its sharp teeth, which can result in the loss of potentially significant amounts of blood – and hence iron – when several hundred or more worms are feeding simultaneously. The presence of hookworms is linked with iron deficiency anemia in a wide range of mostly tropical settings. These parasites, and others, are commonly found in contaminated drinking water where sanitation practices are minimal or nonexistent.

Unlike many other diseases, anemia leaves a definite skeletal imprint that can be observed in dry bones, especially when the disease is chronic. When viewed in X-rays, the marrow space between the outer and inner surfaces of skull bones shows numerous spicules of radiopacity that give a 'hair-on-end' appearance. The space tends to be expanded, the hard outer table of cranial bone is thin, and the area in the tops of the eye sockets is thickened and porous. These changes are due to increased red blood cell production in response to iron losses, and also tend to expose the soft spongy bone in the marrow, presenting a porous bone surface.

The skull pathology is part of a generalized syndrome called *porotic hyperostosis*, a term first introduced in 1966 by the paleopathologist J. Lawrence Angel, who used it to describe the changes he observed in skulls from the ancient eastern Mediterranean – especially ancient Greece. Similar bony lesions found in the upper parts of eye sockets are called *cribra orbitalia*. Clinical and paleopathological evidence indicates that the two conditions, porotic hyperostosis and cribra orbitalia, are caused by the same circumstances that lead to iron deficiency anemia. Therefore, anthropologists who study iron deficiency in ancient populations subsume the two names under porotic hyperostosis.

Porotic hyperostosis has been found in thousands of juvenile and adult skeletons worldwide. Most skulls with active lesions – where there is little or no evidence of bone healing – are found in children of less than five years of age. Most pathology in adults is well healed, indicating an episode or duration of iron deficiency much earlier in their lives. It has been suggested that the different pattern along age lines indicates that for most people the anemia episodes occurred during childhood. This appears to be so because the space between the outer and inner surfaces of skull bones of young children is completely occupied with red marrow, and an increase in activity due to red blood cell production leads to expansion and skull thickening typically seen in porotic hyperostosis. In contrast, adults do not use all available marrow space during increased red blood cell production. Thus, no expansion occurs. Adults may, then, have iron deficiency anemia, but the disease does not leave the characteristic bony changes seen in juveniles.

The record of iron deficiency anemia as it is determined by observations of pathology in skulls is abundant in ancient populations. Fossil hominids bear little evidence of anemia. Not until the Mesolithic period (*c.* 10,000 to 6,000 years ago) following the retreat of glaciers at the end of the Ice Age did noticeable frequencies begin, particularly in the eastern Mediterranean region studied by Lawrence Angel. The most profound increases in pathology occur, however, much later, mostly in the last four or five thousand years, in populations living in permanent settlements.

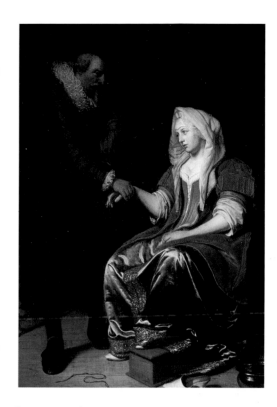

Doctor taking a young woman's pulse. (Michael van Musscher, 1645–1705.)

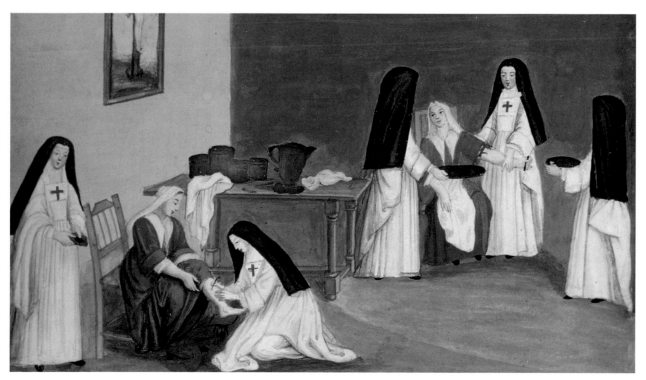

Nuns caring for the sick. (Unknown French artist, eighteenth century.)

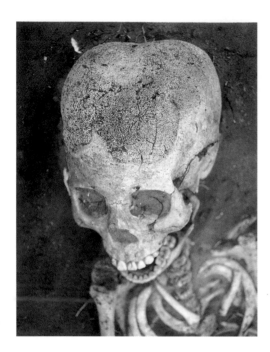

Seventeenth-century American Indian child in Spanish Mission, Amelia Island, Florida, with severe lesions on top of skull resulting from iron deficiency anemia. (Photo by Rebecca Saunders.)

Angel was the first to study anemia in an ecological context using large numbers of skulls from one region. Based on his examination of some 2,200 skulls from ancient Greece, Cyprus and western Turkey, he proposed that the high prevalence of porotic hyperostosis in ancient populations of this area resulted from hereditary anemias, especially sickle cell anemia or thalassemia. In the eastern Mediterranean, where malaria was endemic, individuals who had the genes for sickle cell disease or thalassemia possessed an advantage over individuals with normal hemoglobin. Carriers of the genes for these abnormal hemoglobins showed lower infection rates by malarial parasites (genus *Plasmodium*), and consequently enjoyed greater protection from malaria. Peoples living in the region today do indeed possess relatively high frequencies of abnormal hemoglobin. Moreover, the gene marker for thalassemia has been recently identified in DNA recovered from a child's skeleton from a prehistoric site in Israel. Thus, it is fully conceivable that porotic hyperostosis

in the eastern Mediterranean was caused by a genetic anemia, since the bony changes are not distinguishable from acquired anemia. Other studies of populations from Africa and the Americas indicate, however, that living conditions and lifestyle – non-genetic factors – may be more important causes of anemia in the ancient past.

In the Nile Valley of the Sudan, in the region known as Nubia, scientists found high prevalence (21 percent) of porotic hyperostosis in the Meroitic (350 BC–AD 350), X-group (AD 350–550) and Medieval Christian (AD 550–1400) periods. Reconstruction of possible environmental circumstances leading to anemia, based on archeological, historical and ethnographic evidence, indicates that the disease in this setting was probably related to a number of factors, diets centering too closely on milled cereal grains (wheat, millet), which are foods high in phytates that contain very little iron, along with endemic hookworm disease and schistosomiasis. These circumstances, combined with chronic diarrhea, also highly prevalent in the region today, indicate that the disease was due to acquired iron deficiency anemia. Further to the north in the Nile Valley at Kulubnarti, porotic hyperostosis reached even higher levels, at 45 percent. Kulubnarti juveniles appear to have suffered tremendously: the incidence of the pathology exceeds 90 percent.

In the New World, ancient populations clearly had difficulties with maintaining healthy serum iron levels. In the American Southwest, porotic hyperostosis is highly

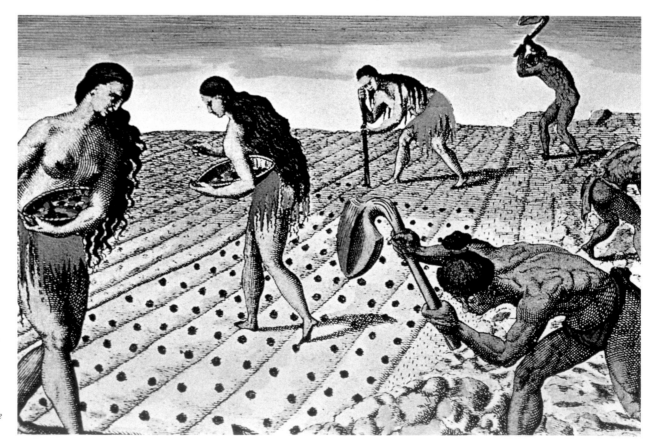

Indians working in maize fields in Spanish Florida during the sixteenth century. Maize is lacking in iron, contributing to iron deficiency anemia. (de Bry, 1591.)

prevalent for many skeletal populations studied by physical anthropologists. At the site of Chaco Canyon alone, scientists found that nearly three-quarters of individuals – 71 percent – had the characteristic skeletal lesions associated with iron deficiency. They concluded this was caused by an over-reliance on maize, a food known to inhibit iron absorption, especially when consumed in large quantities. Study of other New World populations in the American Midwest and Southeast and Canada lends mixed support for this dietary hypothesis. Some prehistoric agricultural societies had high frequencies of porotic hyperostosis (greater than 15 percent), such as those who were late prehistoric maize farmers in the lower Illinois River valley, central Tennessee and southern Ontario. In comparison with early prehistoric populations who were dependent on foraging and collecting of wild foods, agriculturalists had a higher frequency of porotic hyperostosis. At the Dickson Mounds site in Illinois, half the population had iron deficiency anemia.

Prehistoric populations from the Georgia coast have very low prevalence of porotic hyperostosis, probably due to the combined consumption of maize and seafood, which were so readily available to native groups. After the arrival of the Spaniards and the establishment of Roman Catholic missions in Georgia and Florida, the prevalence of porotic hyperostosis rose dramatically, particularly in those groups living around the mission centers on barrier islands. At Mission Santa Catalina de Guale de Santa Maria, frequency of porotic hyperostosis was 27 percent. This represents a tripling in prevalence, which appears to be related to the introduction of the practice of well construction by the Spaniards. Wells represented a new means of acquiring water but, unfortunately, the types of shallow wells dug by Indians were easily contaminated. Moreover, the mission villages were unsanitary, and as a result the overall health of native groups declined precipitously.

Lower social ranks in prehistoric societies may have also suffered more from iron deficiency anemia than higher ranks. In the few comparison studies of populations carried out by anthropologists, low-ranking persons had higher frequency of porotic hyperostosis than high-ranking individuals. Low-ranking female sacrificial victims from Mound 72 at the late prehistoric Cahokia site in western Illinois have the pathology; high-status individuals do not. These differences express a dichotomy in health – at least as it is represented by iron status – in this prehistoric society. This pattern continues to the present day. One has only to travel to Third World countries and observe the deprived living conditions – and presence of iron deficiency anemia – among the poor versus the wealthy.

The increase in frequency of iron deficiency anemia as inferred from increases in porotic hyperostosis in ancient populations may have actually been beneficial. Clinicians have long observed a link between low iron status and decreased microbial invasion, conferring what has been called a type of nutritional immunity. It has been noted that animals and humans not withholding iron are at increased risk of infection (bacterial, fungal, protozoan) and, conversely, risk of infection decreases with increased iron withholding. Pathogens causing infection are dependent on iron that they extract from the host. If the human host is low in iron stores, then the infection declines.

Is iron deficiency anemia – at least in its mild or moderate form – an adaptation to chronic pathogen loads? It may well be. However, iron deficiency anemia carries a direct functional cost, both for the individual and for the population. When a person is even only slightly iron deficient, a number of key enzymes necessary for bodily functions (e.g. DNA synthesis) are affected. Iron deficiency anemia also has profound negative effects on work capacity, cognition and maintenance of a healthy immune system. Nowadays children who are iron deficient perform poorly in the classroom, and usually experience a range of behavioral problems.

Anthropologists are unable to determine the levels of mortality caused by iron deficiency anemia in ancient peoples, largely because anemia is an unusual disease in that by itself it does not lead directly to death, particularly in its mild or moderate form. However, physical anthropologists have found that in ancient populations individuals with the skeletal manifestations of anemia died younger on average than those lacking anemia. Both in present-day and ancient societies, iron deficiency anemia may serve to ameliorate increased infection loads, but it is nevertheless accompanied by other profound health costs.

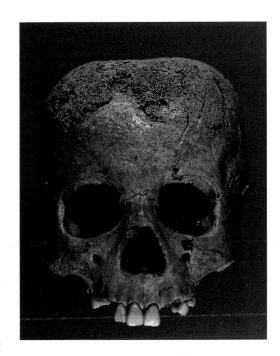

Seventeenth-century Indian child from Spanish Florida. The roughened, porous bone on the top of the skull is a response to severe iron deficiency anemia. (Photo by Mark C. Griffin.)

BIBLIOGRAPHY

Farley, P. C. and J. Foland. 1990. 'Iron Deficiency Anemia: How to Diagnose and Correct', *Postgraduate Medicine*, vol. 87, pp. 89–101.

Goodman, A. H. 1994. 'Cartesian Reductionism and Vulgar Adaptationism: Issues in the Interpretation of Nutritional Status in Prehistory', in K.D. Sobolik (ed.), *Paleonutrition: The Diet and Health of Prehistoric Americans*, pp. 163–77. Carbondale, Illinois.

Larsen, C. S. 1997. *Bioarchaeology: Interpreting Behavior from the Human Skeleton*. Cambridge, England.

Larsen, C. S., C. B. Ruff, M. J. Schoeninger and D. L. Hutchinson. 1992. 'Population Decline and Extinction in La Florida', in J. W. Verano and D. H. Ubelaker (eds.), *Disease and Demography in the Americas*, pp. 25–39. Washington.

Ortner, D. J. and W. G. J. Putschar. 1985. *Identification of Pathological Conditions in Human Skeletal Remains*. Washington.

Stuart-Macadam, P. L. 1989. 'Nutritional Deficiency Diseases: A Survey of Scurvy, Rickets, and Iron-Deficiency Anemia', in M. Y. Iscan and K. A. R. Kennedy (eds.), *Reconstruction of Life from the Skeleton*, pp. 201–22. New York.

Stuart-Macadam, P. and S. Kent (eds.). 1992. *Diet, Demography, and Disease: Changing Perspectives on Anemia.*

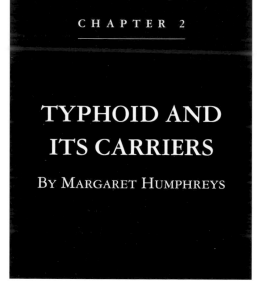

CHAPTER 2

TYPHOID AND ITS CARRIERS

By Margaret Humphreys

Typhoid fever is a classic disease of sedentary life. It probably emerged soon after humans settled near water sources long enough to pollute them, and has been with us ever since.

Although rare in developed countries nowadays, it remains a major world health problem. About 75 percent of the world's population lives in areas where typhoid is endemic and there are 15 million cases and over a million deaths per year.

The symptoms of typhoid fever are so non-specific that we do not know if Hippocrates described it or if Caesar Augustus had it. But, clearly, by the eighteenth century the disease was widespread in Europe. Typhoid fever is caused by a member of the Salmonella family, *Salmonella typhi*. Over 1,700 serotypes of salmonella have been identified, and most have animal as well as human hosts. These include mammals, birds, reptiles, amphibians, fish and insects. Human outbreaks of salmonella infection have been traced to pet turtles, milk from infected cows, eggs covered by salmonella during the laying process, and stuffed turkeys not cooked at high enough temperatures. But typhoid fever is an exclusively human disease, with a protective coat that helps it to hide from the human immune system.

Typhoid fever makes its victims miserable. It is marked by abrupt and prolonged diarrhea (or sometimes constipation), abdominal pain, fever as high as 105 degrees Fahrenheit, blinding headache, cough and severe exhaustion. Often faint patches of rosy red color occur on the abdomen, making the diagnosis more obvious. The fever pattern is one of sustained high temperatures, gradually rising and gradually falling, and sometimes lasting for weeks at a time. Complications, which can be fatal, include pneumonia, intestinal perforation, gastrointestinal hemorrhage and coma. Mortality in typhoid fever ranges from 10 to 20 percent in the absence of antibiotic therapy.

One mechanism by which the typhoid bacillus increases its likelihood of transmission is by the creation of carriers. A carrier is a person who does not appear ill but is capable of spreading an infectious disease. Early twentieth-century studies showed that up to 3 percent of typhoid patients become colonized by the bacteria. Often the bacteria reside in the gallbladder and biliary ducts, whence they are intermittently spread by the unwitting carrier.

The transmission of typhoid fever is technically described as fecal–oral spread, which means that in some way the organism moves from the gut of the infected individual into the mouth of its next victim. This may happen through the fecal pollution of water supplies, such as when the contents of a privy leak through the soil into the water table of a well. The bacteria may travel person-to-person, passing from minuscule amounts of feces on unwashed hands to the hands or food of others, and then reaching the mouth. Flies are effective carriers of typhoid, if their feet touch fecal material and the flies then land on food or someone's face. Those who nurse the sick or wash soiled bedclothes can also get the bacilli on their hands, and hence into their mouths. Typhoid is a disease of poor sanitation. Good sewers, clean water, adequate hand washing and window screens all but eliminate the opportunities for transmission of the disease.

Medicine took a long time to recognize this deceptively simple fact, however. The first problem was that the disease was not easily distinguishable from the many others that cause fever, a rash, headache and gastrointestinal disturbances. Indeed, at the start of the nineteenth century many physicians believed that there were at most a few types of fever, and that all the different manifestations they saw were created by the influence on these core types of climate, gender, race, season and geography. Typhoid was particularly confused with typhus, as their similar names imply. Both were associated with filth, and rightly so. Typhoid spreads best in unsanitary surroundings full of crowded, dirty people; typhus, which is

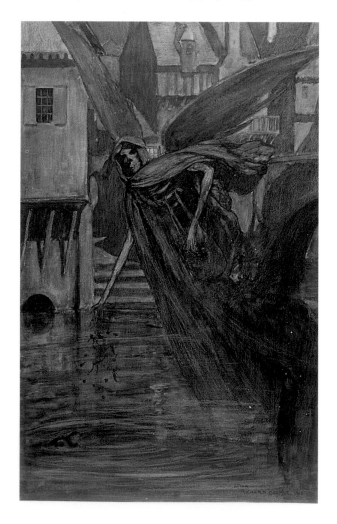

A metaphorical angel of death drops typhoid poison into a town's water supply. (Watercolor, after R. Cooper, 1912.)

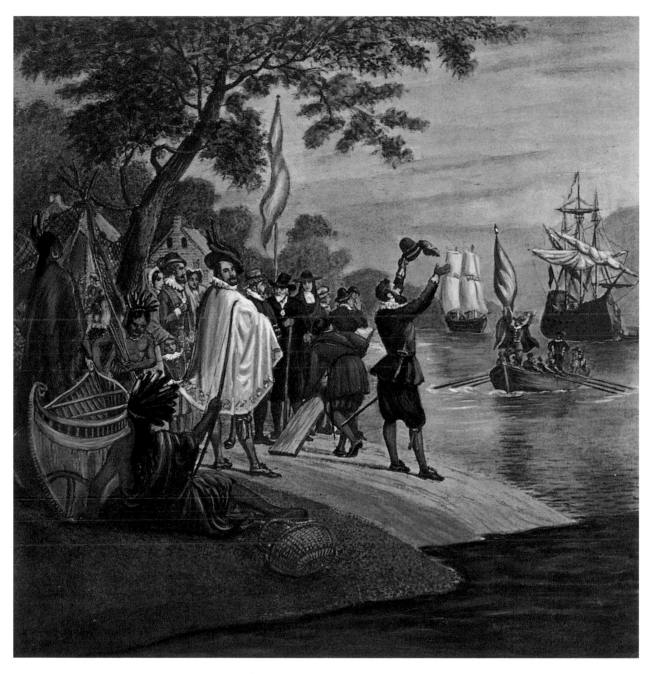

The English land, and found Jamestown, on the low-lying shores of the James River, where the high water table ensured the easy transmission of typhoid. (1607, litho, seventeenth-century English school.)

carried by the human body louse, shares a similar propensity for dirt and poverty.

During the first decades of the nineteenth century this filth theory of disease was elaborated by many physicians in Europe and America. The correlation seemed obvious – as the industrial revolution generated urbanization, more and more people crowded into increasingly dirty cities. Primitive methods of sanitation, relying on privies and wells, were quickly overwhelmed by the rapid growth of population. Overcrowding brought intestinal diseases such as typhoid, as well as pneumonia, smallpox, erysipelas and tuberculosis. No urban physician could miss the explosion of early mortality, and the association with filth came naturally. The theory

argued that it was foul air that made people sick. This foul air might arise from streets filled with manure, dead animals, garbage and fecal material, as well as from diseased bodies lying in the tightly enclosed spaces of the nineteenth-century tenements. Such foul air poisoned the body, generating fevers and debility.

This theory had a lot going for it, for sanitation did improve the population's health. But, as early as 1839, William Budd argued that typhoid did not arise spontaneously from filth, but was on the contrary a contagious disease. After studying an epidemic in North Tawton, England, he felt that it was indisputable that infection had spread from one person to another. From the

Robert Koch (1843–1902),
a country doctor in
Germany, who created the
science of bacteriology.
The identification of the
typhoid bacillus by his
students led to disease
control through water
purification.

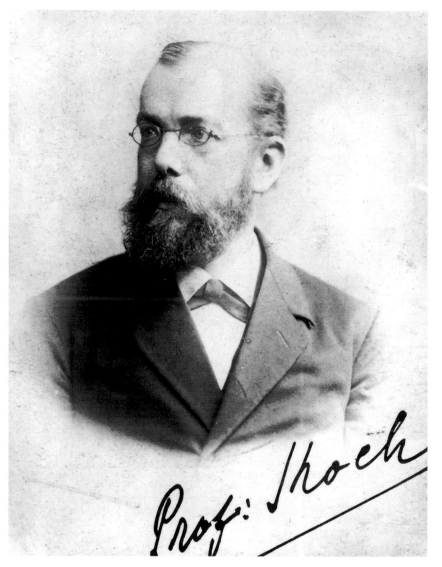

Prof: Koch

fact of contagion he concluded: 'The communication of this fever is effected by means of a material agent, which thrown off from the body of an infected person, produces the same disease in another. This agent is therefore the real and proximate cause of the disease, just as the virus of smallpox is the real and proximate cause of that malady.' In his 1839 essay Budd argued that this agent was transmitted through the air, and also distinguished typhoid from typhus, on the basis of clinical and pathological differences. Although Budd submitted the essay for a prize, it came in second; his readers believed his ideas were a bit too controversial to be awarded first place.

Budd bided his time, and investigated other epidemics of typhoid. In 1847 he was called to the bedside of a fever patient in Clifton, a suburb of Bristol. He discovered a small epidemic of typhoid in the neighborhood, and was surprised to find that what distinguished the afflicted from the healthy was their use of a common well. The case of two academies for girls was particularly striking. One used the common well, and many students became ill with typhoid, while the other had an independent source of water, and none of the girls was sick. Budd expanded his understanding of typhoid's causation to include the possibility that the poison could be spread by water. He finally published this heretical opinion in 1859. Several factors contributed to its receiving a sympathetic hearing. The death of Prince Albert from typhoid, for one, brought the disease to the forefront of the national consciousness. Also, in 1858 a combination of high temperatures and low rainfall created a stagnant, malodorous Thames. In an experiment few would have cared to perform deliberately, the 'sewage of nearly three millions of people had been brought to seethe and ferment under a burning sun, in one vast open cloaca lying in their midst'. Budd cited this experience to prove his point that foul odors alone would not cause illness. 'The result we all know. Stench so foul, we may well believe, had never before ascended to pollute this lower air. Never before, at least, had a stink risen to the height of an historic event.' Day after day, week after week, letters to *The Times* complained of the nuisance, and physicians who believed in the filth theory of disease predicted great outbreaks of pestilence. But oddly enough, the disease rates that year were lower than usual. Budd felt that nothing was clearer than that stinks alone could not cause disease. The poison was specific, had to come from typhoid patients, and travel through the air and water. While acceptance of his conclusions was not immediate, his careful research convinced many readers. By the 1870s it was widely accepted that the poison of typhoid, whatever it might be, was spread by sewage-contaminated water.

Using the microscope and the techniques described by Robert Koch and Louis Pasteur, great progress was made in understanding the causation of infectious disease in the 1880s. One after another, microbiologists established the bacteria that generated tuberculosis, anthrax, pneumonia, diphtheria, cholera and a host of other diseases. Typhoid proved a bit elusive, but was finally captured. In 1880 German researcher Carl Eberth published a description of rod-like organisms that he had found in the lymphatic tissue of fatal cases of typhoid. But he failed to isolate the organism in pure culture, an essential step in the process of proving that a germ is indeed the cause of a disease, and not just a secondary invader or incidental finding. Typhoid bacilli are difficult to grow, particularly if allowed to compete with the common gut organism *E. coli*, since the latter will swarm over the culture plate and obscure the typhoid bacillus. In 1884 G. Gaffky, who worked in Koch's lab, did succeed in isolating the typhoid organism in pure culture, but even then he had trouble generating new cases of typhoid and proving the germ was the causative agent of the disease. Since only humans are susceptible to typhoid, his laboratory efforts with rats and guinea pigs naturally failed. Still, Gaffky and Eberth share the fame of discovering the cause of typhoid. Along with Budd's work on its transmission through polluted water, and the Widal diagnostic test introduced in 1896, public health officials now had the tools to control a typhoid epidemic.

Or so they thought. All that was needed, according to this model, was to disinfect the excreta of typhoid patients, and ensure a clean water supply to the population. Typhoid would fade away as civilization and prosperity brought these basic public health measures. Certainly the typhoid rate dropped, but it did not disappear altogether. In 1901 Koch discovered a disturbing new fact about typhoid: it could be spread by apparently healthy carriers. Although two years earlier American physicians had suggested this might be the case, it was Koch's description of this phenomenon that convinced medical opinion worldwide. He studied eight typhoid cases around the city of Trier. After examining all the contacts of the patients Koch found that seventy-two persons were actually infected with the typhoid bacillus. Fifty-two of those cases were children, although only three had been diagnosed by their physicians as having typhoid .

The most famous typhoid carrier was 'Typhoid Mary'. Mary Mallon was an Irish immigrant who worked as a cook for wealthy New York families in the first decade of this century. She was discovered when one family hired George Soper, a sanitary engineer, to investigate a significant outbreak of typhoid at their Long Island summer home in 1906. Soper at first suspected a polluted well, or a contaminated food source such as milk or cheese. All were examined, and found innocent. Soper had read Koch's paper on the carriers at Trier, and became suspicious of a cook named Mallon who had left the family's house since the typhoid cases developed. Soper tracked Mallon down in her new home, where she angrily refused to give a stool specimen, and denied ever having had typhoid fever. Soper had strengthened his case by tracing her places of past employment, and finding many more typhoid patients in those households, who had contracted the disease while Mallon was there. He got a court order incarcerating Mary Mallon for examination. Her stools were teeming with typhoid bacilli.

What to do? Mallon persisted in denying that she was a threat to anyone. She had her own lab tests done independently, and those results showed no bacteria. This is not surprising in retrospect, for all typhoid carriers shed the bacteria only intermittently. Following a groundswell of popular indignation at her unfair incarceration, Mallon was freed after three years in jail. One condition of her release was that she should keep in touch with public health authorities, nor should she take any jobs as a cook. After trying to sue the city for damages, she promptly disappeared. Five years later Soper found her, working under an assumed name, as a cook in a hospital.

She returned to prison, where she remained until her death in 1938. The Mallon case moved from newspaper headline into the realm of public fable and memory. Even the British joined in the chorus of retribution against her. *Punch* published a satiric poem in 1909, which reflects the anonymous author's anti-Irish sentiment as well as his/her attitudes toward Mary, who 'is just as germy as the day/ On which she went in quarantine'. The poem begins:

'In U.S.A. (across the brook)
There lives, unless the papers err,
A very curious Irish cook
In whom the strangest things occur:
Beneath her outside's healthy gloze
Masses of microbes seethe and wallow
And everywhere that MARY goes
Infernal epidemics follow.'

This hostility was not an isolated reaction. Altogether, Mary Mallon had been responsible for three known typhoid deaths, and at least forty-seven cases, without the slightest sign of repentance or willingness to comply with the restrictions imposed on her. In her wake 'Typhoid Mary' entered our vocabulary as a phrase for any person who wantonly broadcasts disease into a community.

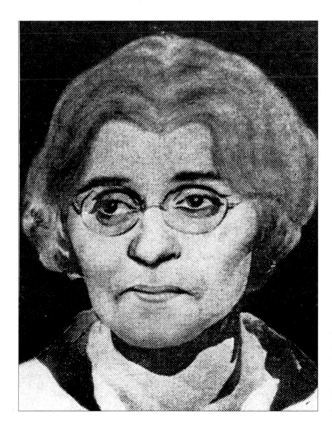

Drawing of the Irish cook Mary Mallon, known as Typhoid Mary, the world's most famous typhoid carrier. (M.D. Medical News Magazine, 1969.)

Anti-typhoid vaccination, World War I.

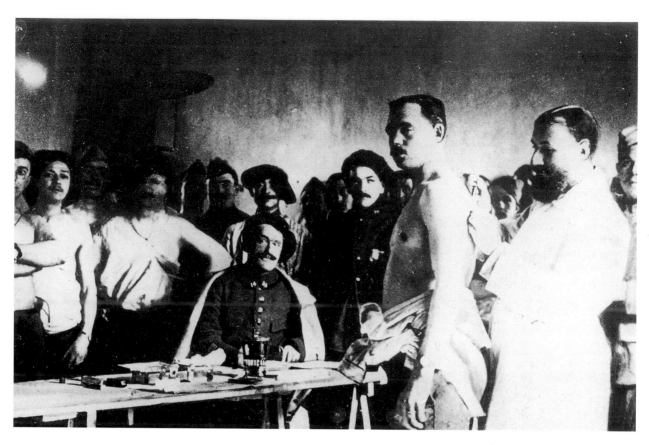

Mallon's situation was not unique. Certainly there were many other carriers in the population, since 3 percent of patients with typhoid go on to the carrier state, in the absence of antibiotic treatment. Charles Chapin of the Providence, R. I. Board of Health summed up this dilemma succinctly in 1918:

'Neither you, nor I, nor the Board of Health, know where these are. The occupant of the next seat may, for all one knows, be a diphtheria carrier … The dirty man hanging on the car strap may be a typhoid carrier, or it may be that the fashionably dressed woman who used it just before was infected with some loathsome disease. If these people were sick in bed we would avoid them. As it is we cannot. Science has shown this new danger.'

Chapin urged that people learn new habits of cleanliness, particularly of washing the hands after going to the toilet and before eating, but also of keeping the hands away from the mouth and eyes. Other public health officials made attempts to track typhoid carriers, especially those who might work in food industries.

Another source of typhoid much dreaded in the early decades of this century was the fly. Insects were newly feared as disease hosts, particularly the mosquito for yellow fever and malaria. But the fly was not limited to country areas or the tropics; here was an insect pest that threatened broad segments of the population. Boards of health called for screens to keep flies away from food, or away from sources of pollution. Cartoons particularly emphasized the threat to

children, with vicious flies hovering over babies, in an attempt to get housewives involved in the anti-fly campaigns.

The newest tool in fighting typhoid in the twentieth century was the vaccine. First efforts to produce one occurred in the 1890s, and by World War I an effective vaccine was available. English and American troops grumbled at being vaccinated for it was well known that it would result in a sore arm. But unlike what happened in the Spanish-American War, when typhoid fever caused far more casualties than bullets did, the vaccinated World War I troops were largely free of this wartime scourge, and this showed that typhoid could be effectively controlled. Since the 1920s typhoid has become a disease of developing countries alone. Communities with clean water supplies deny the organism its principal mode of transmission. Vaccination cuts off the person-to-person contagion that is the second major source of spread. Since the late 1940s antibiotics have been available as well to cure the disease and prevent the creation of carriers. Thus, although typhoid remains a major problem in countries where these aspects of modern medicine and sanitation are too expensive for the public purse, it has largely disappeared from developed nations.

This conclusion is confirmed by public health statistics. The rate of typhoid cases in Europe, North America, Japan and Australia is usually fewer than one case per 100,000 population, with most of these cases imported from endemic countries. A typical story is that of a man born in Pakistan, who emigrated to the United States, where he made his living managing a restaurant. One summer he returned home for a visit, and came down with a case of fever and diarrhea while flying back to Massachusetts. His stool cultures proved positive for typhoid bacilli. After treatment he had to have three negative cultures before officials from the Department of Health would allow him to return to his food production job.

His acquisition of typhoid bacilli in Pakistan was not surprising; there are some 500 to 1,000 cases per 100,000 in South and Southeast Asia, which hosts some of the most severe endemic areas. The combination of poor sanitation and high population density allows the germ to thrive, as it does in the impoverished parts of South Africa (850/100,000), South America (100/100,000 in Chile) and Egypt (40/100,000). Typhoid fever has become a disease of class and ethnicity. It is unlikely that a prince would die of it today. In Israel, for example, the Jewish population has typhoid rates similar to those of the United States, while the Arabs in the area approach the rates of Egypt.

Typhoid fever remains a disease which points the finger at the hygiene of a community. There is a new source of hope, however, with the recent introduction of an oral typhoid vaccine. Unlike the prior vaccine, which caused a sore arm and provided immunity for a few years at most, this vaccine is easy to receive, and may provide prolonged protection. If a solution can be found to the problem of its need for refrigeration, it may offer hope for the ultimate eradication of typhoid fever.

BIBLIOGRAPHY

Budd, William. 1984 (rpt of 1839). *On the Causes of Fevers*. Edited with an introduction and afterword by Dale C. Smith. Baltimore.

Leavitt, Judith Walzer. 1996. *Typhoid Mary: Captive to the Public's Health*. Boston, Massachusetts.

LeBaron, Charles W. and David W. Taylor. 1993. 'Typhoid Fever', in Kenneth F. Kiple (ed.), *The Cambridge World History of Human Disease*. Cambridge, England and New York.

Smith, Dale C. 1982. 'The Rise and Fall of Typhomalarial Fever', *Journal of the History of Medicine and Allied Sciences* 37, pp. 182–220, 287–321.

Stevenson, Lloyd G. 1982. 'Exemplary Disease: The Typhoid Pattern', *Journal of the History of Medicine* 37, pp. 159–81.

Winslow, Charles Edward Amory. 1943. *The Conquest of Epidemic Diseases: A Chapter in the History of Ideas*. Princeton, New Jersey.

Typhoid sufferers on a train in Russia, 1920.

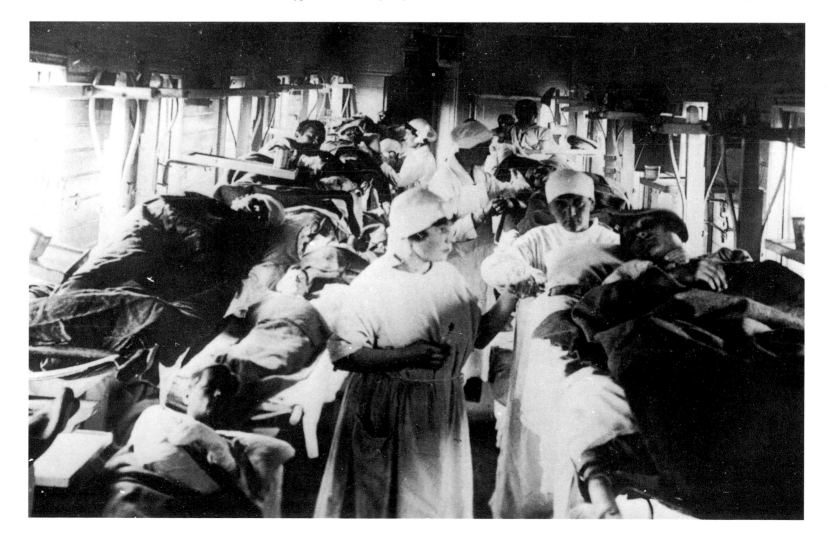

B lood vessels of warm-blooded birds and mammals provide a perfect nutrient-rich environment for a group of parasitic worms, the 'blood flukes', or, to give them their scientific name, the schistosomes. Most of them live in the fine blood vessels of the gut wall, others in those of the bladder and, in birds, some even inhabit the sinuses. In addition all of them, at one time or another, inhabit the veins of the liver.

They all have similar life-cycles, involving passage through snails. The worm eggs pass out of the mammal or bird in either the urine, faeces or nasal discharge and, if they land in water, hatch to produce a very small larval stage, just visible to the naked eye. These larvae must, in the few hours they have to live, find and penetrate into the tissues of a suitable snail. Here they undergo a dramatic asexual reproduction whereby one will multiply to eventually produce multitudes of larvae which are liberated from the snail by their hundreds every single day. These swimming fork-tailed larvae, called *cercariae*, bore back into the bird or mammal host, drop off their tails, and find their way back into the blood vessels where, once again, they produce their eggs.

Fortunately only a few of the schistosome species are human parasites. Of these, three are particularly important: *Schistosoma japonicum* and *Schistosoma mansoni* which are found in the blood vessels of the gut, and *Schistosoma haematobium* which inhabit those of the bladder. *S. japonicum* is an oriental species; it occurs in the Yangtze Valley and some coastal provinces of China and has presumably spread from there to some islands in the Philippines, Central Sulawesi and, at one time, Japan. *S. mansoni* and *S. haematobium* are both African species. The latter is found in most countries of West and Central Africa and from Somalia south to Natal and the Transvaal. It is particularly common in the Nile Valley and Delta, and has also found its way into the Middle East. *S. mansoni* has a similar African distribution and it, too, is very common in the Nile Delta. But, unlike *S. haematobium*, it has found a home in some Caribbean islands and in Brazil, Venezuela and Surinam, having been carried there by the slave trade. Other African schistosomes are sometimes encountered in humans, and in 1978 a new species, *Schistosoma mekongi*, was found to infect people in the Mekong River and Delta.

The worms were not discovered until 1851. A German director, Wilhelm Griesinger, and his assistant, Theodor Bilharz, had just been appointed to the Kasr el Aini Medical School in Cairo. During an autopsy Bilharz found what he later realized was a male and female schistosome worm, and the following year saw larvae hatching from the worm eggs. Ten years later Bilharz died of typhus and his discoveries (although they had been published) were seemingly forgotten.

Egyptian interest in the worms did not revive until the British appointed another German, Arthur Looss, to the Cairo Medical School in the 1890s. It was Looss who initiated a nasty controversy with Patrick Manson and Luigi Sambon of the London School of Tropical Medicine over how many human schistosome species existed in Egypt and their life-cycles. Looss claimed there was but one species there and that its life-cycle was similar to that of the hookworm, which he had uncovered by 1901. In hookworms, and also in schistosomes according to Looss, the larval stage hatching from the egg directly bored back into the human skin. Not until World War I did Robert Leiper, also from the London School of Tropical Medicine but posted to the Royal Army Medical Corps, resolve the controversy by showing that there were indeed two species, *S. haematobium* and *S. mansoni*, that passed through different snail hosts during their life-cycles.

Leiper's crucial discoveries rested, however, on earlier work of Japanese investigators who had first shown the necessity of snail hosts and had observed and described the *cercariae*. A few months after this discovery Leiper arrived from China, where he had been sent to investigate *S. japonicum*, and saw with his own eyes these *cercariae* issuing out of the snails and carrying the distinctive fork tail. Armed with this knowledge he was then able to unravel the life-cycles of the Egyptian worms a few years later.

The diseases which result from these parasites are generally called schistosomiasis or bilharzia, the former named after the genus of worm (*Schistosoma*) and the latter after Bilharz who first saw them. The diseases are caused by the eggs, which, instead of passing out of the human body, become lodged in various organs—the liver, spleen, gut wall, bladder wall, ureters, genital tracts, lungs and even the brain. The diseases do not usually kill, rather trapped eggs set off immune responses with the subsequent appearance of the classic chronic disease symptoms. These include inflammatory lesions around the eggs producing enlargement, obstruction and serious malfunctions of the surrounding organs. In the case of *S. haematobium* a regular and painful discharge of blood occurs when urinating. The seriousness of schistosomiasis depends upon the number and location of these trapped eggs which in turn depends on the host's 'worm load', or the number of worms in the body. Both the prevalence and seriousness of the diseases will be high when the population has an intimate relationship with rivers and canals that are the habitat of susceptible snails.

The diseases have a very complex epidemiology, resulting from an intricate relationship between the parasite and the snail hosts. To simplify somewhat, although the parasites are usually, but not always, capable of infecting quite a wide range of bird or mammal species, each parasite can infect only a very narrow range of snails.

With these facts about the schistosome parasites in mind we can now turn to speculating on the ancient origins of the disease which today is said to infest over 200 million people in seventy-four countries.

In the hunter-gatherer societies of early humans, one can assume that they probably shared their schistosome parasites

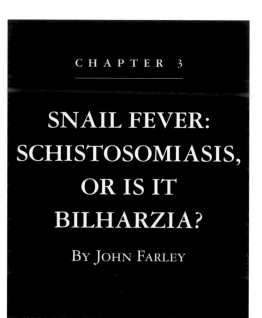

CHAPTER 3

SNAIL FEVER: SCHISTOSOMIASIS, OR IS IT BILHARZIA?

By John Farley

with other mammals, especially primates, as is the case today with *S. mansoni*. But the level of infection would probably have been low, as the only time either humans or primates would have incurred danger of infection would have been during visits to drinking sites that they and the primates would have contaminated with urine and faeces, and where the water would house infected snails. However, when humans began to settle into agricultural societies along river valleys, they would have fulfilled two of the three conditions required for schistosomiasis to flourish: infected humans or other animals and an intimate contact between humans and water. Susceptible snails in the water would have fulfilled the third requirement. As a result human contact with snail-carrying water would have increased and the diseases would have become more of a threat, with a higher prevalence and greater worm loads. These valleys could then become not only endemic sites of schistosomiasis, but also the focus from which the parasites could have been carried along trade routes to other parts of the globe. All these criteria were

met with a vengeance in the Nile Valley where infected people and animals settled approximately 7000 years ago. When joined by susceptible snails, a ready environment for the parasites to undergo their cycles of development was established.

Today no other people on earth suffer the ravages of bilharzia more than the Egyptian peasants, the *fellaheen*. The figures are astonishing: fully 47 percent of the entire Egyptian population were infected according to an estimate of 1937; sixteen to twenty million carried the worms in the opinion of two Egyptian physicians of the 1970s; and modern surveys in villages of the Nile Delta have revealed that virtually all of their children carry the worms. Indeed, so many young boys show the bloody urine characteristic of *S. haematobium*, that it has been popularly regarded as the male equivalent of menstruation.

These high figures have come about because of social and agricultural practices which first became established almost as soon as humans began to settle the Nile Valley and Delta. The

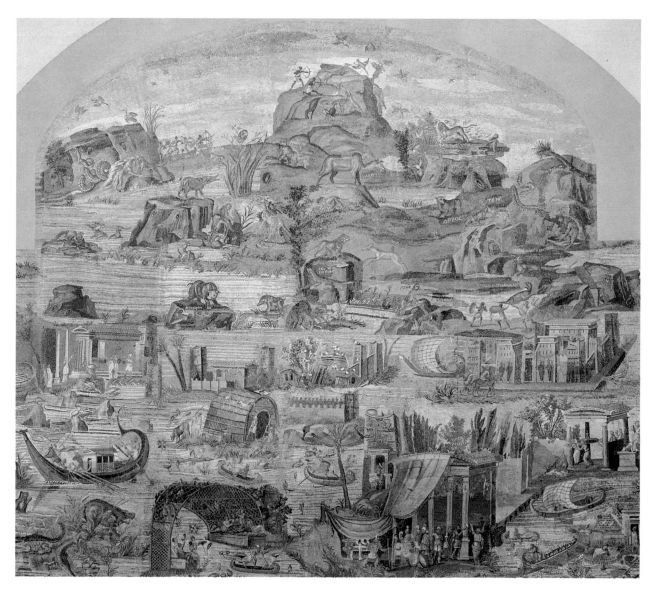

Roman mosaic showing life on the Nile River. (First to second century AD.)

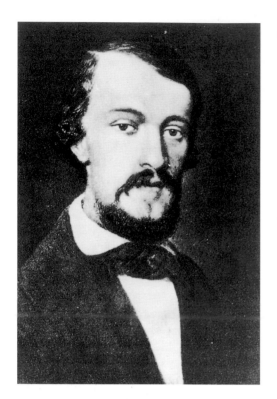

*Theodor Bilharz
(1825–62), who first
discovered the parasitic
worms in 1851.*

fellaheen spent many hours of each day wading in water, which quickly became contaminated with human excrement and parasite eggs. And when the water also became home to susceptible snails, these soon became infected.

At first, large dikes were constructed on both sides of the Nile south of Cairo. These divided the land into a series of basins, some as large as 100,000 acres, and into which every July and August the floodwater of the river was diverted, to stand two to three feet deep, depositing its rich silt into the soil. When the water subsided in November the winter crops of wheat and barley were planted, to be harvested in the spring. In addition water could be lifted into small canals for irrigation by means of a 10-foot-long cylinder with a wooden spiral inside, the ancient Archimedian screw. In such an environment the prevalence of schistosomes and the worm loads may have stabilized at a relatively low rate, because at least in the summer months, when the basin water dried up, the snail–human contact was lost. Today, in areas where basin irrigation is still practised south of Cairo, the prevalence of *S. haematobium* among the villagers stands at about 5 percent, although rates among children are far higher.

This pattern probably lasted for centuries and some, but not all, scholars believe that a disease called *âaâ*, mentioned in sixteenth-century BC Egyptian papyri, may have been due to *S. haematobium*. Whatever the case, calcified eggs of *S. haematobium* have certainly been found in the kidneys of two mummies from the twentieth dynasty of the New Kingdom, traditionally said to have extended from *c.* 1184 to 1087 BC.

In the nineteenth century the agricultural pattern began to change, with the result that the *fellaheen* were forced to spend even more time in water. Especially deep canals were dug in the Nile Delta from which, even in periods when the river was running low, water could still be raised by screws and water wheels to irrigate summer crops, in particular cotton, which soon became Egypt's primary cash crop. Perennial irrigation had arrived and with it came more bilharzia. Contact between the *fellaheen,* water and infected snails now took place on a year-round basis. Modern evidence suggests that when perennial irrigation replaces basin irrigation, the prevalence of bilharzia may increase ten times or even more.

But worse was to follow. The British took control in Egypt in 1882, and soon introduced more agricultural changes. More acres in the Nile Delta were brought under perennial irrigation and British engineers completed the Aswan water-storage dam in 1902 which brought huge tracts of land along the Nile Valley also under perennial irrigation. Thus, at the end of an unsuccessful 10-year attempt to eradicate bilharzia from Egypt (1930–1940), south of Cairo 5 percent of the population were infected with *S. haematobium* in areas of basin irrigation, whereas 60 percent of them were infected where perennial irrigation had been introduced. Similarly, in the Nile Delta, 60 percent were infected with *S. haematobium*, while in the lower reaches of the Delta 60 percent were also infected with *S. mansoni*.

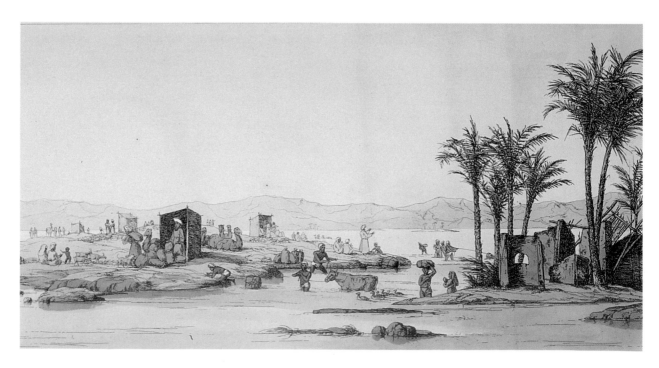

*'Overflowing of Nile,
Egypt', by G. Belzoni,
1822. No other people
suffer the ravages of
bilharzia more than the
inhabitants of Nile
villages.*

The same scenario existed in China. Around 3000 BC millet, rice and barley farming began in the flood-plains of the harsh and unstable Yellow river in Northern China, which required the building of dams, dikes and canals. Bilharzia may have been established here despite the unfavourable environment; a corpse from the second century with evidence of the disease has been recovered. But it was when the Chinese were able to settle and cultivate the warmer and wetter areas around the Taiku, Poyang and Tongtin lakes of the more stable Yangtze river, that the requisites for bilharzia were in place. The Chinese disease associated with *S. japonicum* is generally considered to be the most serious of the schistosome diseases, in that these female worms produce about ten times more eggs than those of the other species which infect humans, and the reaction to these eggs seems more severe.

By the time the People's Republic of China was proclaimed in 1949, over ten million Chinese peasants were estimated to have been infected with the disease, then endemic to eleven provinces along the Yangtze as well as south coastal areas of the country. The havoc wreaked by the disease had become part of Chinese folklore, as, for example, 'The Village of Widows', in Kiangsi Province. There, where acres of potentially productive land had gone to weed, 'scourged by famine, the people survived on seaweeds in spring, wild herbs in summer, husks in autumn, and handouts in winter. Many ended the nightmare of their existence by suicide.' In more recent times, according to Wu Zhili, Surgeon General of the Chinese People's Liberation Army, troops coming down from the north were required to learn to swim in order to do battle in the southern provinces. They did so in the Yangtze, where thousands came down with bilharzia. Military training was suspended and barracks became hospital wards. According to an article in *Harper's Magazine* in 1959, the blood fluke kept Formosa from Communism. In the time taken to build the army back up to fighting strength, the US Seventh Fleet arrived on the scene and the opportunity to destroy the Chinese Nationalists disappeared. Today the disease is still a serious health problem in the Dongting Lake region of Hunan Province, and the construction of the Three Gorges Dam on the Yangtze will inevitably further increase its spread.

Curiously the ancient civilizations of the Indus and Ganges valleys remained free of the disease, and apart from one doubtful and very limited focus of *S. haematobium* in India, that subcontinent today remains free of human schistosomes, although there are many species found in Indian cattle and birds. Luck favored the Southern United States too. Whereas *S. mansoni*, brought from Africa during the slave trade, found susceptible snails in parts of South America and in some Caribbean islands and became established there, closely related snails in the United States have proved to be non-susceptible. Nor are there many mammalian schistosomes in North America, although in much of the lake country of the north, cottage owners suffer from 'swimmers' itch', brought

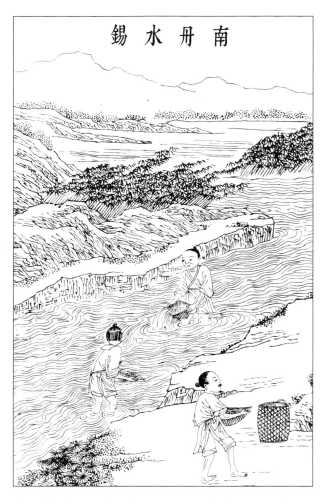

南 舟 水 錫

Where schistosomiasis could flourish. An illustration from a late Ming handbook of Chinese industries showing intimate contact between humans and water.

about by the accidental penetration of the *cercariae* larvae which normally develop only in birds. Once in the skin of some unsuspecting bather, they are quickly destroyed but in the process a tissue reaction sets in, leading to a highly irritating and itchy rash.

BIBLIOGRAPHY

Adamson, P. 1976. 'Schistosomiasis in Antiquity', *Medical History* 20, pp. 176–88.

Farley, J. 1991. *Bilharzia: A History of Imperial Tropical Medicine.* New York.

Farley, J. 'Schistosomiasis', in Kenneth F. Kiple (ed.), *The Cambridge World History of Human Disease.* Cambridge, England and New York.

Jordan, P. and G. Webbe. 1982. *Schistosomiasis. Epidemiology, Treatment and Control.* London.

1977. 'Report of the American Schistosomiasis Delegation to the People's Republic of China', *American Journal of Tropical Medicine and Hygiene* 26, pp. 427–57.

Ross, A. *et al.* 1997. 'Schistosomiasis control in the People's Republic of China', *Parasitology Today* 13, pp. 15–25.

Scott, J. A. 1937. 'The incidence and distribution of the human schistosomes in Egypt', *American Journal of Hygiene* 25, pp. 566–614.

Tien Hsicheng, 1971. 'Schistosomiasis in mainland China. A review of research and control programs since 1949', *American Journal of Tropical Medicine* 10, pp. 26–53.

ANCIENT AILMENTS: MEDIEVAL MALADIES

From the Neolithic revolution to the fall of Rome, humankind was immunologically tempered in a fearsome crucible of disease. This we know with certainty; but it is a theoretical kind of certainty that throws too little light into a dark corridor of human history. One of the reasons we can be certain that this corridor was a pathogenic gauntlet is that today we share some sixty-five diseases with dogs, fifty with cattle, forty-six with sheep and goats, forty-two with pigs, thirty-five with horses, and twenty-six with poultry. It was mostly during these blacked-out millennia that pathogens brought together by a union of people with animals were perishing and prospering, adapting and mutating, evolving from one disease stage into another until they became the plagues that burst upon humankind during the last millennia or two.

Much of the reason for the (apparent) delay in the debut of full-blown epidemics is that many of these evolving diseases would require relatively large and dense populations to support them. But through the mist of time we can occasionally spy previews of what was coming. We know that a plague of terrible proportions struck Athens in 430 BC, but we do not know what it was any more than we know the identity of most of the various biblical plagues. The Roman Empire was staggered during the second and third centuries AD with two epidemics that were said to have slaughtered between 25 and 50 percent of the populations in their paths. Once again, their identities are unknown, although the suspicion has been voiced that they were smallpox and measles (or diseases ancestral to them), appearing in Europe for the first time.

Pathogens suddenly loose among a virgin soil people (those with no prior exposure to them) have been relatively recent phenomena as well as ancient ones; consequently we know something of the mortality that can be generated. When smallpox reached isolated Iceland in 1717, it killed 36 percent of its people. When measles struck nineteenth-century Hawaii and the Fiji Islands for the first time, it eliminated a quarter of those populations. When Indian groups in the Amazon rain forest have been discovered and, consequently, suddenly exposed to the disease environment of the outside world they have sometimes died out completely. And there are estimates of the catastrophic population collapse of the Native Americans following the introduction of foreign pathogens after 1492 which suggest

a die-off of 90 percent or more before population recovery began.

These modern-day demographic disasters (relatively speaking) are mentioned to help us grasp something of the magnitude of the ordeal our ancestors were subjected to as their immune systems were painfully developed. The dense populations required by many illnesses took shape only gradually, but by around 3000 BC, centers of 50,000 or more inhabitants had arisen in Mesopotamia and Egypt, closely followed by others in the Indus Valley. Individuals in populations where a particular disease arose generally developed resistance to it. But restless humans – marauders, missionaries, merchants and the like – did not leave those populations in isolation for long, with the result that people were regularly exposed to newly introduced diseases against which they had no resistance. Massive mortality ensued (perhaps of the order of 90 percent), followed by painful demographic recovery that, in turn, was followed by still more massive die-offs as one people's familiar disease became another people's plague.

It was only by around AD 1200 that much of this pathogenic reign of terror came to an end because of the development of what American historian William McNeill has termed a 'confluence of disease pools', meaning that by this time people throughout the Old World had come to share immunities to the same epidemic illnesses. But increased use of the products of domesticated animals and an even greater reliance on grains fostered still more new diseases. Moreover, as populations grew and people were more closely packed together, they became increasingly easy targets for diseases of wild animals against which they could not possibly have gained any immunity. And, finally, it was during this transition from a mystical to a modern world that attention was focused on mysterious diseases that people seemed to be born with – perhaps at the behest of gods or God – but affected only relatively few individuals.

The chapters in this section are intended to illustrate all of these points and to continue the theme of progress as a disease-causing agent. For example, the progress that opened trade across the Indian Ocean brought the Plague of Justinian to the Mediterranean world of the sixth century. This may have been the first excursion of plague into Europe although as we will see later on, it certainly was not the last. Plague had such devastating effect because humans had developed

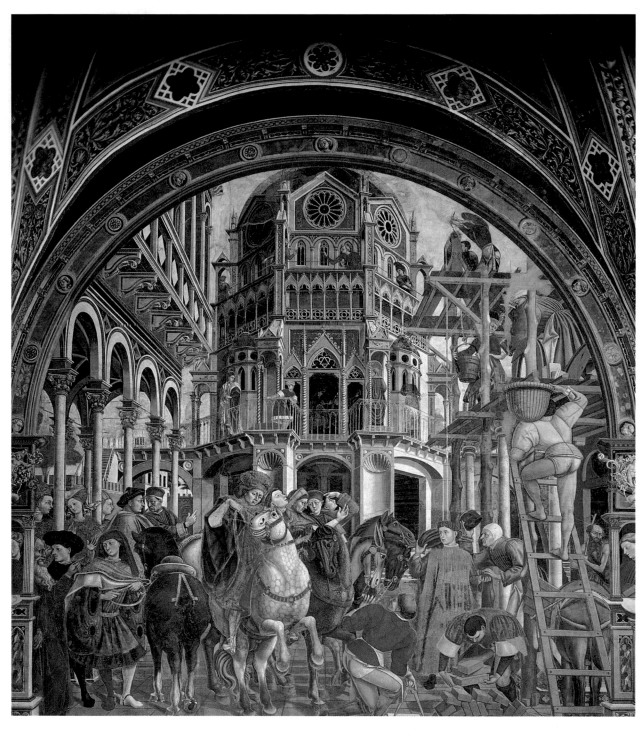

Construction of hospital fresco by Domenico di Bartolo, 1443, Santa Maria della Scala Hospital, Sienna.

no immunities against it as it is a disease of rodents and their fleas, with humans only accidental victims.

We have already noted that the progress of the Neolithic revolution, which promoted population growth, also narrowed the human diet considerably and forced a concentration on cereals. This situation, which continued into the Middle Ages, proved deadly for many consumers of rye, who frequently consumed along with it a toxic fungus on the rye. The disease ergotism was the result. Yet another disease that came with agriculture was scrofula, a kind of tuberculosis caused by using dairy products from cows sick with this disease.

The progress that led to urbanization was also most likely responsible for leprosy which may be identified in the Bible. What is a fact is that societies, and the religions they create, have tended to stigmatize victims of diseases such as leprosy and epilepsy – a condition also treated in this section.

Bubonic plague, a disease of wild rodents and their fleas, is most likely an ancient one. But how long it has accidentally affected humans is less certain. Perhaps 'incidentally' is a better word than accidentally because, in a cycle widely believed to be the method of transmission of all plague epidemics that struck Europe, rat fleas carry the causative bacillus *Yersinia* (formerly *Pasteurella*) *pestis* to the common black or brown house rat (*Rattus rattus*), that came to be known also as the ship rat and the plague rat. As the disease kills the rat, the fleas abandon it, preferably for another living rat, but if none is available, a human will do temporarily. As the flea bites its new host the disease is transmitted (incidentally) to a human rather than to the rat that nature had designed to receive it.

The homeland of plague is generally thought to have been along the Himalayan borderlands between India and China where it was (and is) perpetuated in rodent populations, although nowadays there are other plague reservoirs as well. But it is generally believed that in the sixth century plague somehow escaped the Asian confines of its cradle and marched westward to slaughter the peoples of the Middle East, North Africa, the Roman Empire and western Europe. It was from Justinian, then Emperor of the eastern portion of the Roman Empire, that the plague took its name. But we are getting ahead of ourselves and ahead of the historical and epidemiological circumstances in which this plague first appeared.

Just as Rome and its Empire had not been built in a day, the Empire had not fallen apart in a day. But it had come apart – cloven into Latin and Greek halves. Although there were numerous reasons for this, two of the most important were assaults by the Germanic kingdoms of western Europe, on the one hand, and devastating onslaughts of pestilence, on the other. This is not to imply that Rome had been especially salubrious prior to this point. Malaria seems to have been ubiquitous, and numerous other diseases frequently hammered the Empire. The Roman historian Livy (59 BC–AD 17) recorded many epidemics during the Republican period and 30,000 people were said to have died in Rome during an epidemic of AD 65. But the plagues that struck the Empire during the second and third centuries were extraordinarily devastating. This was most probably because they were new diseases, against which the population was immunologically defenseless, and, unfortunately for all those vulnerable people, they were also protracted plagues. The first – the so-called Antonine plague – hit the Roman Empire between AD 165 and 180, apparently reaching the Mediterranean with troops returning from the Parthian Wars in Mesopotamia. (Rumor had it that a too-enthusiastic soldier breaking open a casket in the temple of Apollo at Seleucia had released the pestilence.)

The returning soldiers had doubtless been exposed in Mesopotamia to any number of illnesses and the Antonine plague may have been comprised of several of them. However, August Hirsch, the nineteenth-century German epidemiologist and historian, voiced his strong suspicion that, regardless of the number of intertwined illnesses, by far the most important one was smallpox (or a disease ancestral to it), making its first European appearance. Whatever the identity of the pestilence it was so extraordinarily lethal that it was credited with killing between one-third and half of the people in affected areas. A mournful chronicler wrote (apparently with little exaggeration), that everywhere there was desolation. Towns were empty, fields unworked, and estates deserted. In fact, it was this pestilential outbreak that is said by historians to have initiated the general decline in the population of the Mediterranean which continued for several centuries.

Such a decline was surely hastened by the second wave of pestilence. This one washed over the Roman world in 251 and did not fully abate until 266. Again, there are few clues to its identity, although the American historian William McNeill speculates that perhaps this plague, in tandem with its predecessor, announced the arrival of both smallpox and measles in Europe. In any event, this epidemic was at least as deadly as the Antonine plague and at its height it is believed 5,000 people a day were dying in Rome.

Prolonged and bitter civil war, as well as invasion, added to the death toll generated by this second epidemic. One result in this third century of the Christian era was that the Roman imperial government was transformed into a military

---

CHAPTER 4

THE PLAGUE OF JUSTINIAN: AN EARLY LESSON IN THE BLACK DEATH

By Kenneth F. Kiple

This gold denarius (an ancient Roman coin) shows the head of Emperor Justinian (c. 483–565).

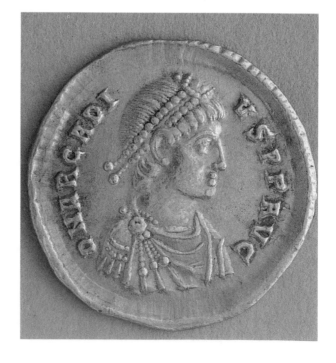

despotism. Military power was exalted above all else to assure the defense of the frontiers and to maintain internal order; and one suspects that mobilization of sharply diminished manpower required despotic measures. The death of Diocletian (285–305) plunged the Empire into another round of civil wars that were finally suppressed by Constantine the Great (306–37). Constantine, of course, is remembered mostly as the emperor who gave Christians complete freedom of worship. But he also moved the capital of the Roman Empire to a 'second Rome' at Byzantium, which was promptly renamed Constantinople, and in 395 the Empire was formally split into two.

The eastern part, economically more vigorous and sufficiently compact to make defense easier, endured (but not without travail) until 1453, whereas the Western Empire was completely overrun in the fifth century. But for a brief moment the Greek portion of the Empire under Justinian (527–65) was poised to bring its Latin counterpart back into the fold. Justinian's administrative reforms, codification of Roman law, and construction of the church of St Sophia were achievements fully matched by his military exploits. He launched a series of campaigns into the western Mediterranean which saw northern Africa, Italy and a part of southern Spain reconquered. Unfortunately for his aim of re-establishing the unity of the Roman Empire, disease, which had so disrupted that Empire in the past, once more took a hand when the Plague of Justinian struck in 542.

The cause of this epidemic can be positively identified thanks to numerous accounts including that of Byzantine historian Procopius of Caesarea who, in his *History of the Wars*, described in detail the course of the epidemic and the symptoms that it produced. In fact, it was his dramatic account of this pestilence that prompted naming the plague after Justinian. Others also described it, including Bishop Gregory of Tours in 1547, as the epidemic surged into western Europe; and many more had the opportunity to write their own agonized versions as the disease ricocheted around the Mediterranean for the next two centuries.

Hirsch called this epidemic the first evidence of 'bubo-plague' in Europe, and bubos are, as the name bubonic implies, one of this plague's tell-tale symptoms. Once a person

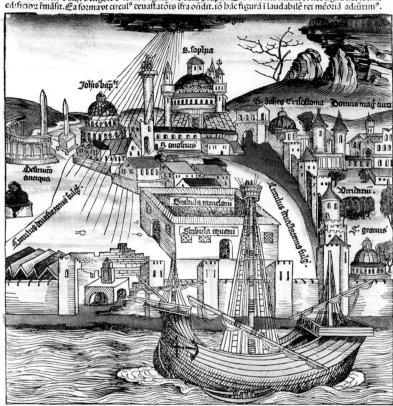

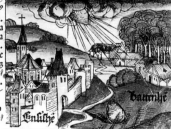

is infected with *Y. pestis*, the lymphatic system tries to collect the infection in lymph nodes and these frequently swell to the size of an egg (or an orange or even a grapefruit), into what was called a bubo. Because fleas usually bite an exposed area of the body, such as the limbs or the face, these bubos, which developed in the nearest nodes, were often visible.

Yet bubos do not invariably appear. The infection can also move so rapidly that it becomes 'septicemic', or blood-borne, and overwhelms the lymphatic system. If the disease reaches the lungs and victims cough out the pathogens, the plague can become pneumonic. In this form the disease bypasses rats and fleas and moves directly from human to human. The account of Procopius hints that the Plague of Justinian did,

View of Constantinople (now Istanbul) on the Bosporus in the late fifteenth century. The scene depicts public buildings including St Sophia in the background, converted into a mosque with the Muslim conquest.

Roman statue of Asklepios (Asclepius), the god of medicine, with staff with serpent entwined; and Hygieia, goddess of health, with Telesphorous, the tiny god of convalescence, at her feet. (Relief, 5th century AD.)

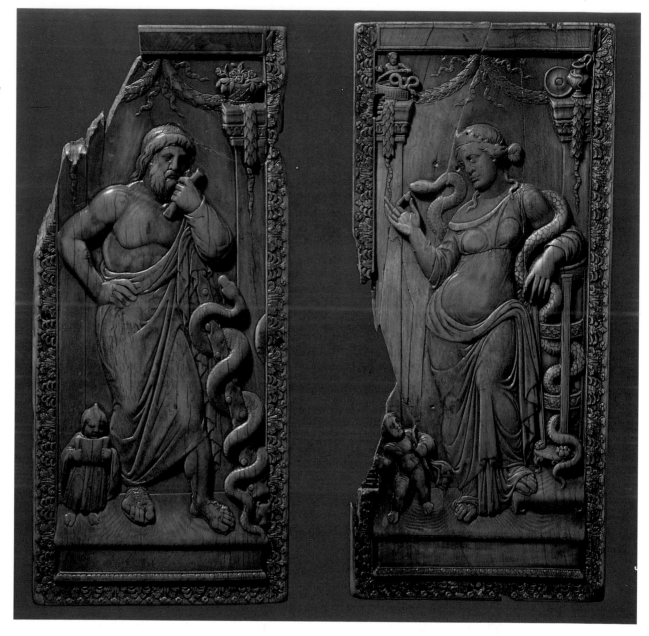

in fact, assume pneumonic form, which, in the absence of antibiotics, would almost invariably have proven fatal.

Although the Plague of Justinian endured only briefly (from 542 into 543), it is generally viewed as the beginning of the first cycle of plague which lasted until somewhere around the middle of the eighth century. Yet, plague was already very much alive long before it struck Constantinople. Procopius placed the beginning of the pandemic in Egypt, and Hirsch points out that Rufas of Ephesus wrote of a disease that struck Libya and Egypt much earlier – in the third century – which (complete with bubos) seems also to have been very plague-like.

The assumption that both of these examples were, in fact, bubonic plague on the move seems reasonable enough. Trade had opened between India and Egypt, and the homeland of *Rattus rattus* – so important in carrying the disease – appears

to have been India, as we hinted at earlier. In other words, the bacillus and its hosts and vectors may well have all migrated together westward out of South Asia.

Although the Romans had established trade and travel across the Eurasian land mass, one suspects that most of the traveling done by the plague rat was aboard ships. Rats are good climbers – *R. rattus* especially so – and the lines that made ships fast to wharves provided a convenient method for boarding in one port and disembarking in another. In this fashion the rats probably fanned out to the cities and towns along the shores of the Indian Ocean and worked their way up the Red Sea to Egypt – all the while establishing colonies as they did so. Rats being good breeders, those colonies probably grew larger and larger until a conduit was opened for *Y. pestis* to pass along stretching from its source in northeastern India all the way to the heart of the Middle East.

Europe lay just beyond, and from Egypt the next leg of their journey would have carried the migrating rats to the port cities of the Mediterranean, eastward through the Dardanelles to Constantinople on the Bosporus, and westward toward the Iberian Peninsula. Then, when the rats (and their fleas) were in place, *Y. pestis* began a sustained trek northward from lower Egypt. Because the *R. rattus* probably had the ability to infect local rats, this may have dramatically increased the risk that humans in its path would become infected.

The onset of this first cycle of bubonic plague was probably as catastrophic as that of the Black Death – the name bestowed on the initial onslaught of the second cycle of plague eight centuries later. In Constantinople it burned with fearful intensity for four months during which, at its peak, Procopius reported that it killed 10,000 persons a day. Justinian himself contracted the disease but was one of those lucky enough to survive. His plans for restoring imperial unity, however, did not. The plague shattered them by sharply reducing the manpower available for more Mediterranean adventure.

Yet this may have been a blessing in disguise because the Mediterranean had suddenly become an extremely insalubrious region to frequent. The plague, which had surged first across its eastern end, next moved westward, rolling over Italy and reaching at least as far as southern France, all the while ravaging the Middle East and North Africa. Surveying the carnage wrought in the Mediterranean, Hirsch quoted an observer who wrote that the plague 'depopulated towns, turned the country into a desert and made the habitations of men to become the haunts of wild beasts'.

The disease is said by some to have stretched also northward to the British Isles in 544 and to have returned there later in the first cycle of plague (in 664), when it was

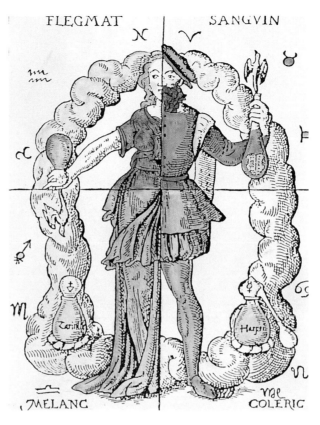

'The Four Temperaments'. 16th-century woodcut.

chronicled by the Venerable Bede, allegedly making yet another appearance in 682. Because Britain lay outside of the plague's Mediterranean trajectory, some have questioned whether bubonic plague actually made any, let alone all, of these early appearances in England. It is the case, however, that islands are extremely vulnerable to imported diseases, and certainly the British Isles were linked to the Mediterranean. Moreover, since it seems clear that England was indeed assaulted by outbreaks of pestilence while plague was raging, it makes sense to suspect that the pestilence in question was plague. And finally, that some disease(s) potent enough to bring about demographic decline (like plague) did strike England seems borne out by the fact that in the centuries that followed its population was at a surprisingly low level when compared to continental countries that we know were not visited by the first cycle of plague.

Overall, mortality was placed by contemporary observers at 100 million (a number that must have defied calculation in Roman numerals), and although this may seem steep for the first few years of the plague such a guess may not be too wildly off the mark for mortality resulting from the two centuries that the plague persisted. It is generally accepted that the first cycle of plague did claim at least 25 percent of the population of the two Roman Empires, whatever that number may have been. And it is worth noting for comparative purposes that the Black Death was later credited with killing between 25 and 50 percent of the populations it visited in both Europe and the Middle East.

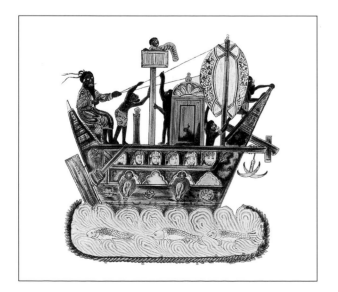

Arabic ship, spreading plague as it moved from country to country.

Some groups would have suffered more than others. People in rural villages had the best chance of escaping plague completely. The inhabitants of rat-infested port cities, where the rodents were constantly coming and going with visiting ships, would have been directly in its path. Inland urban dwellers would also have been at considerable risk because their cities were havens for rats, and because the chances of plague assuming its very lethal pneumonic form were best among closely packed populations. That the first cycle of plague did not penetrate into northern Europe suggests that *R. rattus* had not yet finished its migration in that direction, although it seems possible that it had reached the British Isles by sea, and was on hand to first host and then spread the disease there.

The political, economic and social effects of the plague rippled outward over many centuries to come. As a demographic disaster of the first magnitude, it not only ruined Justinian's plans for reuniting the eastern and western portions of the Roman Empire but it so weakened the Roman and Persian armies that they were helpless in the face of the Muslim military might that spearheaded the expansion of Islam,

beginning in 634. Moreover, as McNeill has pointed out, 'the perceptible shift away from the Mediterranean as the preeminent center of European civilization and the increase in importance of more northerly lands …' was another result of this and other epidemics that followed.

But perhaps most significant of all, it would seem that the Plague of Justinian, and the two centuries of plague that followed, marked the end of the Classical World and the beginning of the Dark Ages. In the wake of this pestilence came diminishing trade replaced in most places with little more than barter economies; cities withered and feudalism grew; religion became intensely fatalistic, and Europe shrank into itself.

Numerous mysteries surround this first cycle of plague, by far the biggest being the question of why the disease vanished from Europe for almost 600 years after its last mention in Christian sources in 767. Surely, the rats were still in place. Could it be that the accepted notion of a migration of *R. rattus* touching off the disease in the first place is not a valid one? It is true that this rat is not normally a migratory animal, and nowadays relatively few are found in Europe outside of port

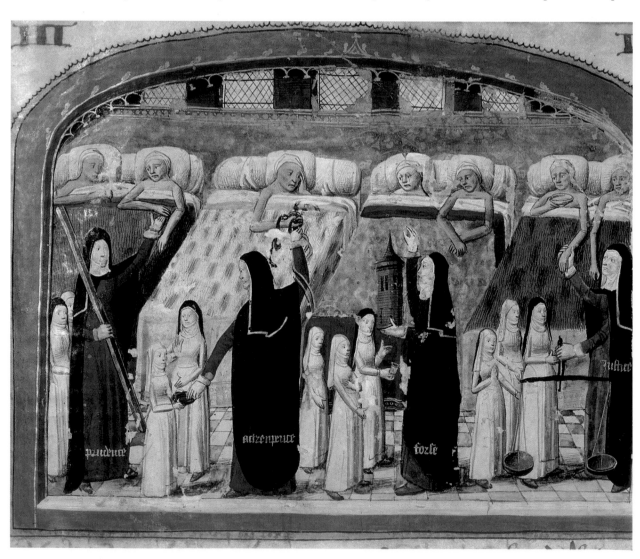

'Musée de l'Assistance Publique.' Sick patients in a ward at the hospital Hôtel de Dieu, Paris, from Livre de la Vie active, *by Jean Henry, 1482.*

cities. Nor was there any mention in the admittedly scanty literature of the Plague of Justinian and its sequelae of 'rat falls' – the explosive black rat mortality that so often signalled the appearance of plague elsewhere in later times. Could it be that the disease reached Constantinople by way of infected fleas but not the rats?

The development of human immunity against the plague can be ruled out as an explanation of the disease's disappearance. Surviving the plague may have conferred some short-term protection, but even persons in our own era who are vaccinated against it have to be revaccinated frequently. Could the rats have developed an immunity to *Y. pestis* that broke the cycle of transmission?

Rodents other than the black rat can also carry the plague, and one, *Rattus norvegicus*, probably did help to spread the disease in later centuries. This Norwegian rat is larger and more aggressive than the black rat and may well be the reason why so few of the latter are found in Europe today. Its migrations throughout Europe, however, took place hundreds of years after the first cycle of plague had ended.

There is, of course, always the possibility that *Y. pestis* did not actually disappear from Europe but instead, after a savage beginning, settled down to become a much milder disease. However, if that is true, why did plague roar back to life after several centuries in a subdued state, to decimate populations with a voracious appetite for close to half a millennium?

The most logical, although not entirely satisfactory explanation, hinges on the retreat of Europe into itself while the first cycle of plague first raged and then wound down. This is because, for reasons that remain enticingly obscure, *Y. pestis* apparently never achieved what is called a sylvatic or enzootic foothold in western Europe. It did not, in other words, establish the kind of permanent presence that it had managed in the Himalayan borderlands between India and China amidst rats and other rodents, and that it has subsequently achieved in Central Africa and the western United States; in fact, almost everywhere in the world except western Europe.

This, in turn, means that plague had always to be imported, as it was during Justinian's time, when the Mediterranean was open to intercourse with the larger world. But with the first cycle of plague Europe withdrew into itself, and Muslim imperialism assured that such a withdrawal would be a lengthy one. Arab conquests unified all of Arabia and, by 715, had brought the whole of the Middle East (save for Asia Minor) under Muslim control, along with the lower Indus Valley, North Africa and the Iberian Peninsula. Clearly, Europe was not only besieged, but effectively cut off from the trade and from the plague, which flowed from India.

Nor was there much European energy to devote to expanding ties with the wider world. In addition to seemingly endless wars internally, Europe was regularly threatened with invasion from the east. These threats culminated in the Mongol conquests and the mounting pressure of the expanding Ottoman Empire. It seems to have been these advances, uniting so much of the known world, that also reunited Europe with the plague.

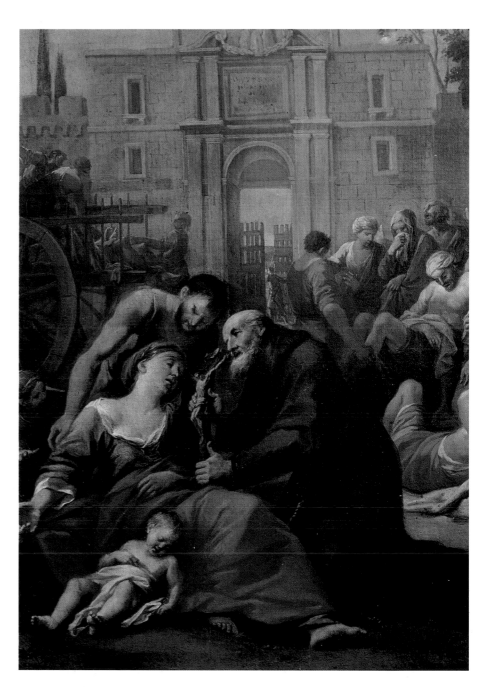

BIBLIOGRAPHY

Carmichael, Ann G. 1993. 'Bubonic Plague', in Kenneth F. Kiple (ed.), *The Cambridge World History of Human Disease*. Cambridge, England and New York.

Hirsch, August. 1883–6. *Handbook of Historical and Geographical Pathology* (tr. Charles Creighton), 3 vols. London.

Jackson, Ralph. 1988. *Doctors and Diseases in the Roman Empire*. Norman Oak and London.

McGrew, Roderick E. 1985. *Encyclopedia of Medical History*. New York.

McNeill, William H. 1976. *Plagues and Peoples*. Garden City, New York.

Winslow, Charles Edward Amory. 1943. *The Conquest of Epidemic Disease* (1980 reprint). Madison.

Cardinal Chigi heals plague-ridden people in Rome. (Artist unknown. Palazzo Barberini, Rome.)

ERGOTISM AND ERYSIPELAS: ST ANTHONY'S FIRE

BY KENNETH F. KIPLE

'St Anthony's Fire' was a frequently described disease-condition in Europe during the Middle Ages. Nowadays scholars can be reduced to guesswork when trying to find for it a name with medical meaning. In most cases St Anthony's Fire probably meant ergotism – a disease that August Hirsch, the great German epidemiologist of the nineteenth century, listed as epidemic some 130 times in Europe between 591 and 1879 while, at the same time, acknowledging that these occurrences probably represented just a tip of the proverbial iceberg.

In other instances, however, St Anthony's Fire signified recurrent erysipelas. Other names, such as 'hidden fire', 'saint's fire', 'evil fire', 'holy fire', 'devil's fire' and *Ignis* (or *Ignes*) *Sacer* (sacred fire), also add to our already considerable confusion and, even worse, it is generally acknowledged that at one time or another St Anthony's Fire was probably a name for everything from wound infections to the plague and from scurvy to smallpox. By the same token, however, if diseases called St Anthony's Fire were many things besides ergotism and erysipelas, we can at least be reassured, in sorting through a pastiche of past pestilence, that outbreaks of erysipelas and especially ergotism, were in fact, consistently called St Anthony's Fire.

Ergotism is a form of fungal poisoning caused by the ingestion of the ergot fungus (*Claviceps purpurea*), which can form on cereal grains, especially on rye ears, and infect the porridge and breads made from the grain. The disease takes two forms. One, called *convulsive*, afflicts the central nervous system, whereas a second, *gangrenous*, form affects the cardiovascular system by constricting arteries and veins that deliver blood to the extremities. The disease has exterior symptoms such as reddening or blistering skin, which presumably were seen as manifestations of the fire in question. Certainly, the gangrenous form of the disease was another.

In the list of epidemics provided by Hirsch, most that took place between 591 and the fourteenth century did so in France. In French monastic hospices where the sick were cared for, the disease acquired patron saints to whom victims appealed for help. Foremost among them was the Egyptian anchorite St Anthony (c. 251–356).

Alternatively called St Anthony of Thebes, St Anthony the Great, as well as the Hermit and the Egyptian, he is credited with founding Christian monasticism by living a solitary life in the desert where he constantly did battle with the devil. Although a hermit, he became legendary, and expeditions were organized to locate him and seek his advice. He hated such fame and asked his disciples to keep his burial place secret when he died. Apparently they did, but 200 years

St Anthony of Egypt, the patron saint of those afflicted with St Anthony's fire, with his characteristic symbols of pig and bell.

later by divine revelation, according to legend it was discovered and he was reburied in Alexandria. A century after this, however, St Anthony was moved again, this time to the church of St Sophia in Constantinople. There he rested for 400 years, until a French Crusader, the Count of Dauphiné, got permission from the Emperor of Constantinople to relocate him once again. In 1070 the Crusading Count, carrying the relics of St Anthony, returned home to the Dauphiné region of France.

St Anthony was not left in peace, however. Almost as soon as his well-travelled bones were laid to rest, healing miracles began occurring that were attributed to his presence. The relics of St Anthony quickly became part of a pilgrimage site established for sufferers of the 'fire'. Next came a hospice operated by friars of the blue Tau – the large Greek letter that came to symbolize St Anthony. He became the most important of the patron saints invoked against ergotism, and the disease acquired his name.

There was, however, a second St Anthony, this one a Portuguese Franciscan monk – St Anthony of Padua (1195–1231). Born in Lisbon, he became a noted preacher in both Italy and France. There he developed a reputation as a healer and all-purpose wonder-worker just as the bones of the first St Anthony were gaining fame and the cult of St Anthony was spreading from France to central Europe and

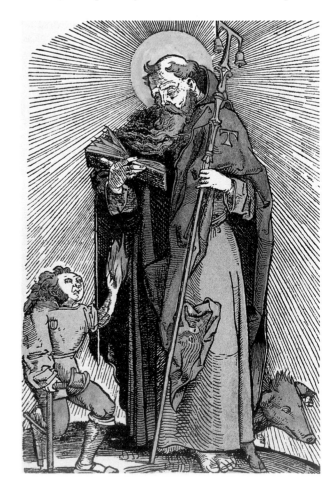

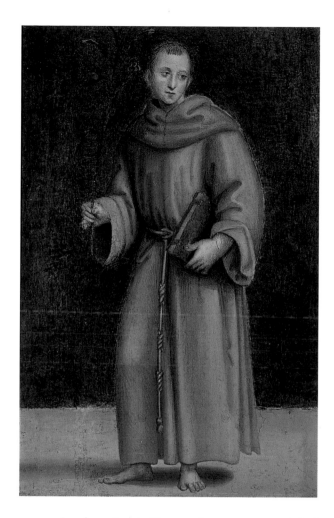

caused the disease. It was a sickness of the countryside – so much so that some physicians referred to ergotism as *morbus ruralis* and of the poor, especially after crop failures or during a famine. It was also a malady of growing children who ingested more food than adults per unit of body weight, and consequently, more of the ergot poison. In addition to rural huts the disease frequented urban orphanages, foundling hospitals and prisons.

Because the ergot fungus grows best in damp conditions, epidemics were most likely to occur after a severe winter, that reduced the resistance of the grain, and a rainy spring, or when rye was planted in marshy land, such as that which is newly cultivated. Wetness is the reason why the French districts of Sologne and Dauphiné – subjected to frequent flooding – were so plagued by the disease. But from at least the eighteenth century until the end of World War II, it was the Russian people, forced by the cold climate to depend on rye – a hardy grass – as their dietary staple, who suffered most from fungal poisoning. The earliest diagnosed epidemic in Russia took place in 1785–6, but that country's literature from the fifteenth through the seventeenth centuries contains frequent references to epidemic nervous disorders and to widespread gangrene – significantly, often associated with famine. In the nineteenth century ergotism was extraordinarily widespread in Russia during the years 1832, 1837 and 1863–4, and in the twentieth century in 1909, 1926, 1928–9, 1932, 1933 and 1938. To single out just one year, 1933 – which saw a very wet spring and summer – as many as 75 percent of the rye ears were infected in some parts of the country. Without a steady increase in potato production and consumption throughout the twentieth century, ergot poisoning would have been even more widespread and the situation even more disastrous. In the absence of dependable mortality data, we cannot even guess at the death toll, but it is worth noting that ergot toxins can pass through mother's milk to poison nursing infants and that at the turn of the twentieth century Russians suffered the highest rates of infant mortality in Europe.

Hirsch was puzzled by the phenomenon of ergot poisoning producing gangrenous disease in some regions such as France, but the convulsive kind in others such as Russia and Germany. Subsequent research, however, seems to have resolved the problem by showing that the difference in symptoms depended most on which alkaloids were produced by a particular *Claviceps* strain. In the convulsive form of the disease the central nervous system is affected when ergotism causes the degeneration of areas of the spinal cord. Anxiety, vertigo, noises in the ears, sensations of being bitten or pricked, even stupor, were among its many symptoms. Often the limbs contracted convulsively, which produced staggering, twitching and other uncoordinated movements. Another symptom was the psychosis that ergotism can produce because ergot alkaloids contain hallucinogenic properties. (In fact, LSD can be extracted from the basic ergot alkaloid.) Most victims recovered, but

St Anthony of Padua, from the Colonna Altarpiece (oil on panel) by Raphael (1483– 1520).

eastward as far as Russia. Because the common people had difficulty distinguishing between these miracle workers, the two St Anthonys were frequently blurred and became something of a composite to whom those suffering from the 'fire' offered up their prayers.

Certainly, victims of ergotism needed all the divine help they could get. In 922 an outbreak of the gangrenous type in France was reported to have claimed 40,000 lives, whereas another, in Paris alone, during 1128–9 killed some 14,000 people. Data gathered during ten epidemics in nineteenth-century Russia revealed that between 11 and 66 percent of those who fell ill died, with a mean mortality rate of 41.5 percent.

Early theories about the cause of ergotism implicated butterflies, worms, even the cooking of the sexual parts of plants. But by the nineteenth century much was known about the disease, and the name, St Anthony's Fire, no longer had meaning, save as a quaint reminder of Middle Ages superstition and obscurantism. In summarizing knowledge of ergotism, Hirsch wrote that its area of distribution was small and that in Europe historically it had been mostly confined to France, Germany and Russia. He added that these were areas which used much rye and that there was no doubt that grain, contaminated with ergot,

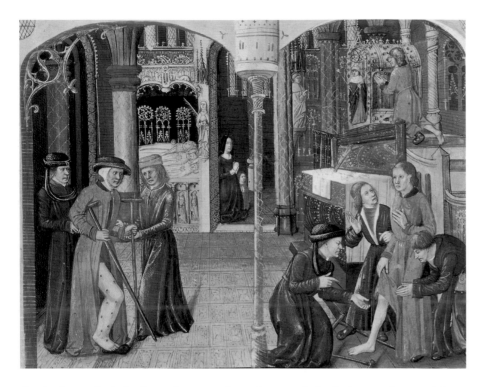

A miracle cure by St Louis (1214–70) of gangrene of the leg.

often not for a long period of time and not without lingering stiffness in the joints, optic disorders, even severe mental impairment.

One interesting example of the historical implications of convulsive ergotism is discussed by Mary Kilbourne Matossian

in the context of the Salem witchcraft trials of 1692 in North America which, following an explosion of accusations and confessions, saw the arrest of some 250 persons suspected of witchcraft and the execution of nineteen of them – five men and fourteen women. The 'bewitched' were children and young women who were thought to have symptoms of diabolical possession but which most likely were those of ergot poisoning. Was rye produced in Salem Village and other parts of Essex county in the late seventeenth century? Yes. Was there ergot in the rye? Ergot produces a red color in bread and three Essex county women who attended a witch sacrament declared that their sacramental bread was red. What symptoms did those allegedly bewitched display? Twenty-four of the thirty victims experienced 'fits' and hallucinations along with the sensation of being pricked or bitten. Others reported feeling a burning in the fingers, lameness and temporary blindness.

Three of the afflicted died, along with several cows, the animal deaths easily explicable as the result of ingesting wild grasses infected with ergot. At the very least, the animal as well as the human deaths suggest that something was going on in Salem and Essex county. It cannot all feebly be put down, as in the past, to suggestible children and teenage girls feigning symptoms which some die-hards believed were evidence that Satan was at work. The youth of the victims may be another clue when we remember that, as a rule, the young will consume more food and consequently more ergot per unit of body weight than adults. Moreover, it is also the case that adolescents are especially susceptible to mental disturbances from ergot poisoning.

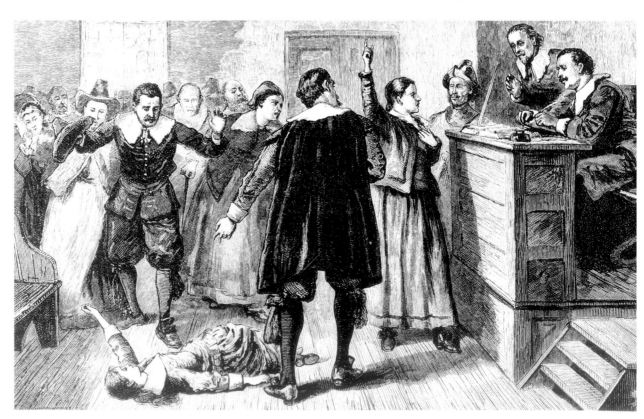

Witchcraft trials at Salem village, 1692. Undated engraving.

Other evidence shows that winters were turning colder and that much of the land planted in Salem was low-lying and wet – all conditions in which ergot grows best. So, Matossian makes a good case that an outbreak of ergotism lay behind the Salem witchcraft accusations of 1692. This opens the door to the possibility of ergot's deadly mischief having been at work in other religiously charged historical situations.

We have selected two examples from the many Matossian has provided; separated by time and geography, to see if they can be linked by ergot. In the first, it is easy to sense the sinister building of epidemic ergotism. The severe winter of 1517 in western Europe was followed by an outbreak of gangrenous ergotism in Strasbourg. During the 1520s the weather was very wet in Germany and then, after another severe winter in 1534, a great number of people began to experience hallucinations and convulsions in the Anabaptist city of Münster. Such symptoms were not, however, confined to Münster but also prevailed among Anabaptists in other cold and wet regions where rye was cultivated, and epidemics of bewitchment had become almost commonplace.

The second example focuses on England where the middle of the seventeenth century was characterized by religious hysteria, such as that exhibited by the Quakers, but certainly not limited to them. During their meetings some Quaker men but mostly women and children fell into fits of quaking and also manifested other strange symptoms indicative of central nervous system derangement. At about the same time other religious groups in England and on the continent had similar experiences with outbursts that seemed epileptic, with exhibitions of spasms, tremors, hallucinations and panic.

While not discounting the suggestibility of some people, Matossian points out (and this is the link) that such behavior was common in an area that included rye-growing Scotland, England, France, the Low Countries, Germany, and the northern parts of Italy and Spain, but it was uncommon in Wales, Ireland, and the central and southern portions of Italy and Spain – areas where little or no rye was grown – and in Scandinavia where cold summers discouraged ergot formation.

Historical research conducted in the 1930s finally resolved the paradox of the different manifestations of ergotism, with the convulsive kind reigning in one locale and the gangrenous type in another. The study of a 1770 epidemic of gangrenous ergotism on one side of the Rhine and convulsive ergotism on the other revealed that the community which experienced the gangrenous kind was a dairying economy whereas the other was not. This, in turn, led to laboratory experiments in which it was discovered that the vitamin A in dairy products was efficacious in keeping the convulsive kind of ergotism at bay because phytase and bowel bacteria are stimulated to break down the poisonous phytates in the grain. Such findings led to the hypothesis that England's relative freedom from convulsive ergotism was attributable to a diet rich in milk, butter and cheese.

To discuss gangrenous ergotism, however, we must go back to St Anthony's Fire. This form of ergotism led to a permanent decrease in the caliber of the arterioles and,

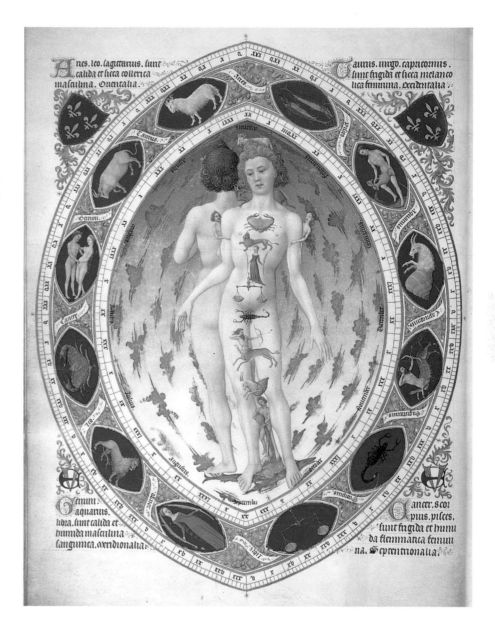

eventually, to dry gangrene of the extremities – usually fingers and toes, but sometimes the ears and nose. It generally began with an itching of the feet and perhaps the sensation of ants running around on them (formications), followed by a burning pain and, perhaps, blisters, and by a spreading 'erysipelatous' redness. The affected area sooner or later would blacken, but frequently sufferers were saved by the removal of the affected parts. Because of the erysipelatous redness, however, in the Middle Ages the afflicted were also frequently said to be suffering from the 'fire'.

Just as Hirsch, writing in the latter part of the nineteenth century, knew a great deal about ergotism, he also knew much about erysipelas. In fact, he discussed it along with puerperal or 'childbed' fever just at the time that medicine was discovering that both were streptococcal infections, whereupon 'erysipelas grave internum' became a form of puerperal fever. However, in also discussing erysipelas in

'The Anatomy of Man and Woman' from the Très Riches Heures du Duc de Berry *(early 15th century). Musée Conde, Chantilly, France.*

terms of what he called 'hospital gangrene', Hirsch perpetuated the ancient error of subsuming gangrenous afflictions with erysipelas.

Erysipelas, as we know it today, is classic cellulitis – an acute disease of the skin and subcutaneous tissue which can produce painful red skin lesions called *peau d'orange* because the human skin assumes the texture of an orange rind. The term erysipelas (*erythros* = red, *pelle* = skin) was used in the days of Hippocrates (*c.* 460–375 BC) to describe the affliction. But confusion crept in because the term was also applied to other skin disorders and at the beginning of the Christian era the confusion became complete. Celsus (*c.* 25 BC–AD 50) lumped together gangrene, skin afflictions and *Ignis Sacer*, and the famous scholar, scientist and physician of second-century Rome, Galen of Pergamum (*c.* 130–200), although distinguishing between classic cellulitis and gangrene, regarded both as erysipelas. Gangrene, erysipelas, ergotism and a host of other ailments all became either erysipelas or *Ignis Sacer*, and later, St Anthony's Fire.

Scarlet fever, also called scarlatina, caused by the same streptococci that trigger erysipelas, was doubtless also given membership in this group from time to time. Its initial symptoms are those of a streptococcal sore throat and it was called by such names as *rossalia*, *purea epidemica maligna* and *febris milaria rubra* – all suggestive of the symptoms of erysipelas.

Interestingly, Hirsch wrote of a 'Remarkable Series of Epidemics in North America' that began in 1822–36 and grew into a pandemic which did not end until the beginning

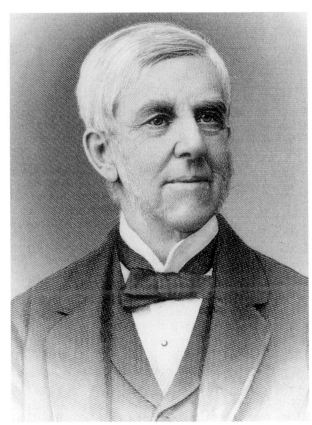

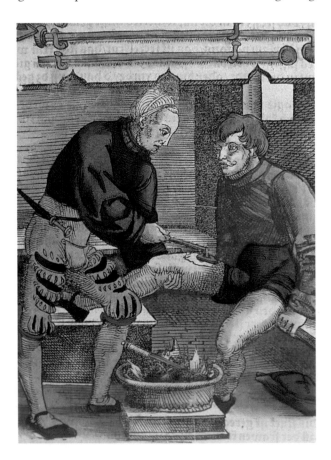

of the 1860s. He called the disease malignant or typhoid erysipelas and declared these epidemics 'with complications of severe throat affection' to 'constitute one of the most interesting episodes in the history of erysipelas'.

Hirsch counted seventy epidemics in all, some of which endured a year or more. The states that suffered the most were those in the west: Illinois, Indiana, Missouri, and parts of Tennessee and Iowa although Michigan, Wisconsin and the Minnesota Territory were also pummelled. However, he mentioned that at times the disease appeared only in hospitals, which means a final detour in this nosological maze.

As already mentioned, the organism that causes what we know as erysipelas today also causes scarlet fever and puerperal fever. Until the end of World War II and the advent of antibiotics, these pathogens were frequently carried in the nose or throat by a large percentage of healthy people who were asymptomatic carriers. In the nineteenth century erysipelas began to receive considerable scientific attention because of epidemics like those just discussed and because these epidemics coincided with peak years of puerperal fever (now more accurately described as puerperal sepsis). Indeed the disease was reportedly responsible for a mortality rate of between 5 and 20 percent of all maternity patients in the larger hospitals of Europe, and when smaller medical facilities experienced outbreaks, fully 70 to 100 percent of the new mothers perished. Clearly, hospitals were very dangerous places to give birth, and outbreaks were not only frequent but on the increase. While acknowledging that it was far from complete, Hirsch put together a list of 195 epidemics that took place between the years 1664 and 1879, nearly 75 percent of which dated from the nineteenth century.

In 1795 Alexander Gordon, an Aberdeen physician, became the first to associate erysipelas with puerperal fever, and by the first decades of the nineteenth century the suspicion had arisen that both diseases were contagious. Among those harboring this suspicion was the American physician and author Oliver Wendell Holmes (1809–94). In a seminal article published in 1843, he described a case in which a physician had examined the body of a man who had died of gangrene of the leg one day and the following day attended a woman who was giving birth. She, and six other women he had treated, developed puerperal fever.

At about the same time that Holmes published this essay, Ignaz Semmelweis (1818–65) became an assistant at the Vienna maternity clinic. There were two wards, one staffed by midwives, the other by medical students. He was puzzled by a maternal death rate of about 10 percent in the students' ward compared with about 3.5 percent in that of the midwives. Following several months of investigation, he became convinced that the disease was transmitted by medical personnel from autopsied and dissected corpses to patients, and he introduced the procedure for medical practitioners of handwashing in a chlorine solution to sterilize them before approaching the sickbed. The results were impressive. The maternal death rate fell to less than 2 percent in his ward. His colleagues, however were not only not impressed, they were outraged at Semmelweis for suggesting that they, who were devoted to healing, could be agents of death. In the face of this hostility, Semmelweis resigned and moved to a hospital in Budapest.

There, in 1861, he published a major book on childbed fever in which he demonstrated that physicians who accompanied their dead patients to the autopsy room, and then returned to live patients in labor lost considerably more of those patients than did midwives who did not perform autopsies. Perhaps it was the furore and controversy that his book stirred up which led to his admittance to a mental hospital in 1865. Ironically it was discovered in the hospital that he had developed an infection in one of his hands that subsequently spread throughout his body and killed him. Semmelweis died of erysipelas caused by the same pathogens that transmitted puerperal fever – the disease he had struggled to conquer.

Fortunately for medicine, Semmelweis was soon vindicated. In the 1860s the French chemist Louis Pasteur's work on sepsis in surgery was applied by others with now predictable, but then astounding results, and in 1879 Pasteur identified the streptococci responsible for causing erysipelas as well as puerperal and scarlet fever. Such nineteenth-century investigations have given us our modern definitions of erysipelas and separated it completely from ergotism – the true St Anthony's Fire.

BIBLIOGRAPHY

Carmichael, Ann G. 1993. 'Erysipelas', in Kenneth F. Kiple (ed.), *The Cambridge World History of Human Disease.* Cambridge, England and New York.

Carmichael, Ann G. 1993. 'Saint Anthony's Fire', in Kenneth F. Kiple (ed.), *The Cambridge World History of Human Disease*, Cambridge, England and New York.

Carter, K. Codell. 1993. 'Puerperal Fever', in Kenneth F. Kiple (ed.), *The Cambridge World History of Human Disease.* Cambridge, England and New York.

Hirsch, August. 1883–6. 'Ergotism and Erysipelas', *Handbook of Geographical and Historical Pathology* (tr. Charles Creighton), 3 vols. London.

Matossian, Mary Kilbourne. 1989. *Poisons of the Past.* New Haven and London.

Ignaz Phillip Semmelweis (1818–65) investigated the causes of childbed fever, the results of which were published in 1861, causing a major furore in the medical profession.

A barber surgeon tending a peasant's foot, c. 1650. Panel by Koedyck (Koedijck) Isaac (c. 1616/18–68).

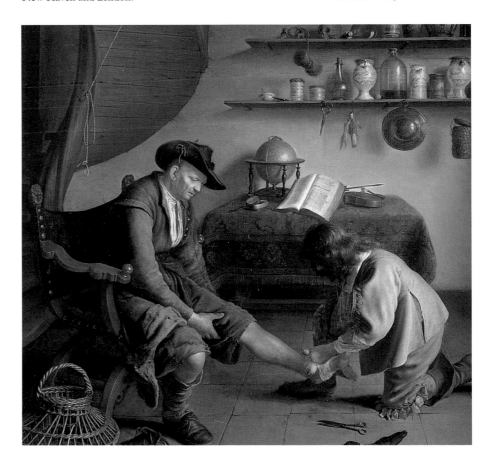

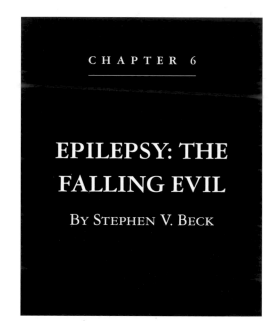

CHAPTER 6

EPILEPSY: THE FALLING EVIL

By Stephen V. Beck

The ancient Greeks called it the 'sacred disease' or the 'great disease'; the Arabs (perhaps translating from the Greek) termed it the 'divine disease'; medieval Europeans named it the 'falling evil' or 'falling sickness'. The disease was epilepsy, a chronic illness still not fully understood by modern medicine, although it has been known to humans throughout history and has been responsible for much misery.

Epilepsy is perhaps best thought of not as a specific disease but as a collection of symptoms. Epileptics are subject to repeated uncontrollable seizures or fits that are nowadays believed to be the result of abnormally large and disjointed electrical discharges by groups of brain cells. Most victims fall down, lose consciousness and fail to remember what happened during an attack. Such behavior is common to all forms of epilepsy, but a variety of other symptoms may occur as well, and their presence or absence and degree have been used to classify different types of epileptic seizures.

Even ancient descriptions refer to these other symptoms: violent movement of the head and neck, fixity of the eyes, tension of the limbs and extremities (even partial and/or temporary paralysis), frothing at the mouth, biting of the tongue, convulsions, and loss of control over bodily functions. Many victims also had an 'aura' (from the Greek word for 'breeze') warning them that an attack was imminent. This sensation might take many forms – dizziness, nausea or faintness, among others – but was described by one second-century AD patient as a feeling that began in the lower leg and gradually rose to the head; when the 'breeze' reached the head, the seizure began. Other auras have involved more bizarre symptoms, such as strange odors or even visions,

but all portended the epileptic fit. Our forebears noted that such symptoms did not necessarily all occur in every case, nor was epilepsy the cause of every fit that anyone experienced. But a seizure of this type coupled with impairment of the sufferer's mental and sensory functions served as an important diagnostic criterion that helped to separate epilepsy from other convulsive or hysterical illnesses.

Possibly the earliest known mention of epilepsy is in an Akkadian text produced by the people who ruled much of Mesopotamia (present-day Iraq) around 4,000 years ago. This text listed some of the symptoms of the illness, which it called *antasubbû*, and referred to its negative moral implications, among them, perhaps, that the sufferer was possessed by demons. Another early document, a Babylonian tablet from about 650 BC, also described epilepsy.

In the ancient Greek world, both Heraclitus and Herodotus mentioned the disease, although the earliest existing extended discussion of it is in a somewhat later work, *On the Sacred Disease*, a medical text probably penned by Hippocrates or one of his followers around 400 BC. The word 'epilepsy' itself comes from a Greek word meaning 'seizure' or 'attack'; this term for the condition appears to be very old, and medical men had already established it in this usage by the time of the Hippocratic writings. But to laymen it was the 'sacred disease' because popular beliefs held that it was caused by demonic possession, or that it was inflicted by the gods (or required a god to cure it), or that it chiefly attacked sinners. Clearly, these ideas stressed its supernatural, rather than natural, character, and, in the face of such popular opinion, the ancient Greek physicians used 'epilepsy' only to mean the attacks or symptoms; the illness itself was still the 'sacred disease'.

On the Sacred Disease, however, argues that epilepsy is not 'sacred' but natural, and should be treated naturally. The author relates the symptoms and progress of the illness, and recognizes it as having a peculiar identity. He states that it is a disease of the brain, most likely hereditary, and further, that all mental diseases result from problems of the brain. He disparages the incredible multitude of popular superstitions and taboos about epilepsy, reviling especially the activities of so-called magicians who claimed to be able to treat or cure the condition. One of the most popular – if gruesome – supposed magic cures for epilepsy was to drink human blood, preferably fresh. Later on, in Roman times, epileptics would enter the arena during the games to drink fresh blood straight from the wounds of injured gladiators.

For the Romans, epilepsy was *morbus comitialis* (the 'disease of the assembly'). According to the third-century AD physician Quintus Serenus, Roman tradition claimed

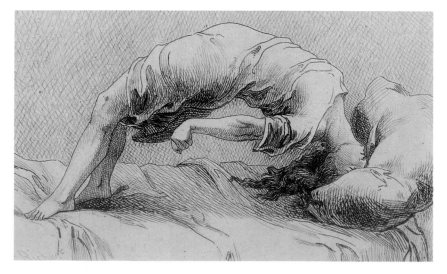

A mental patient at Salpétrière, 1885, showing contortions. From Paul Richer, La grande hystérie. *By 1850 it was standard practice to segregate epileptic patients in insane asylums.*

that, over the centuries, epileptic fits had frequently interrupted the *comitia*, or assembly of the people, thus disrupting the proceedings and hindering the counting of votes. Many Romans, too, saw in epileptic attacks the work of some demonic possession or sorcery, and, as in Greek society, this was disputed by physicians, who nevertheless had little knowledge of what constituted effective treatment. As a rule, treatment centered on diet and regimen.

Despite their shortcomings, the physicians of both Greece and Rome may be credited with wonderfully accurate descriptions of epilepsy, and modern research has in many instances only confirmed their observations. The disease was thought to be most common among children and adolescents. Although it could persist in adult life, it was rare that it struck an adult who had not had attacks when younger, most victims experiencing their first seizure before reaching their majority. Young children or elderly people might be killed by a first attack. But the usual course of epilepsy was chronic, beginning in childhood and growing worse throughout the victim's lifetime.

Although the ancients recognized that the disease was not necessarily life-threatening, they believed that it could permanently affect the physical and mental state, or the personality, of chronic sufferers, causing them, for example, to lose physical coordination or to become extremely confused or unsociable. These ideas are generally rejected by modern medicine, which finds that the effects of a seizure are not permanent and that epileptics, when not actually in the throes of an attack, are usually quite normal in thought and behavior. But there is no reason to doubt the accuracy of the ancients' reporting, for antisocial or abnormal behavior on the part of epileptics in olden times may be explained by factors other than their illness.

In classical antiquity mental disease was believed among laymen to be unclean. Epilepsy in particular was seen as both frightening and possibly contagious. Superstitious Greeks and Romans would spit when they encountered epileptics; the spitting was supposed to keep the contagion (or the demon)

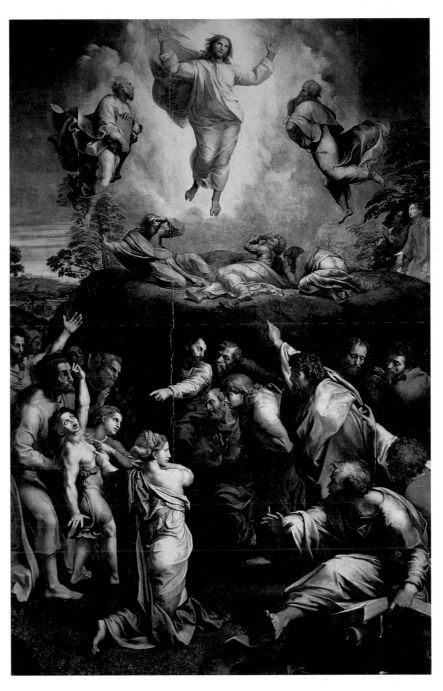

Raphael's painting, 'The Transfiguration', 1517, depicts in the foreground a boy having an epileptic seizure. The incident was described in the Gospel according to St Matthew.

at bay. There is also some evidence that people feared to share dishes or drinking vessels with epileptics. But, most importantly, people who suffered from epilepsy were made to feel acutely embarrassed and disgraced, and tried to hide themselves when they anticipated an attack. The disease signified sin, and, in the eyes of onlookers, the hiding behavior indicated fear and guilt. It is not surprising that in such an atmosphere an epileptic should begin to appear unfriendly or uncoordinated, but this was not a symptom of the disease – it was a reaction to a hostile society.

Although the classical physicians had a fairly clear idea of the symptoms and clinical progress of epilepsy, their

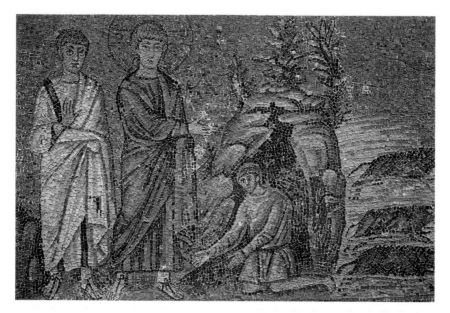

Christ heals the man posssessed by the Devil. Mosaic from the cycle in St Apollinare Nuovo in Ravenna, 6th century AD.

theories about its causes were limited by their lack of medical knowledge. There is some indication that certain later Greeks – notably Asclepiades, Herophilus and Erasistratus – tended to think in terms of the brain and nervous system. We do know that some of these men studied human anatomy, but unfortunately much of their work is lost. Soranus, a Roman physician of the early second century, was perhaps the last for some time to think about epilepsy in this way, because later in the century Galen developed a 'humoral' theory of epilepsy that was so influential that it survived at least through the seventh century. Humoral medicine believed the causes of all diseases lay in the various quantities, imbalances, and mixtures of the body's 'humors' – phlegm, blood and bile. The epileptic seizure itself was caused by the reaction of these substances to climate and other influences, resulting in a thick, 'cold' humor that accumulated in the brain and blocked communication with the rest of the body.

One outgrowth of the humoral theory was a popular belief that the humors of great men made them unusually susceptible to epilepsy. In later times it would be said that, among others, Hercules, Julius Caesar and Mohammed, the founder of Islam, had suffered from epilepsy, but such claims have to some extent been disputed.

In the early Middle Ages popular superstition still ascribed epilepsy to demonic possession, but, in addition, the disease began to be equated with insanity. The seventh-century Bishop of Seville, Isidorus, tells us that an epileptic was called *lunaticus*. Theophanes Nonnus, a tenth-century physician of the Byzantine Empire, still felt it necessary to argue well over a thousand years after *On the Sacred Disease* was written that the disease was the result of bad physical auras or humors and to ridicule the belief that it was caused by demons.

Learned opinions of epilepsy in the Middle Ages were not unlike those of classical times, and exhibited a similar dichotomy. In general, physicians asserted that the disease was natural, but medical knowledge had not advanced much beyond that

Treatment of a headache with a plantain root. (Italian book illustration. First half of the thirteenth century.)

of the ancients. Opposing the medical view was one of religious mysticism, largely repeating – now in the Christian terms of actual bodily possession and exorcism – the classical belief that seizures were the result of demonic or divine influence. These views, however, were able to coexist for some time, for a new element had crept into the debate: the idea that 'natural' seizures (resulting from epilepsy) and 'supernatural' seizures (resulting from demonic possession) both had some validity; the trouble was that it was very difficult to tell the two apart.

Like the ancients, medieval physicians thought that epilepsy might be contagious, and as late as the year 1400 a medical text included epilepsy in a list of infectious diseases. Treatment was still based on the old humoral system, and its effectiveness was doubtful. Much more popular was religious healing. In western Europe, St Valentine became the 'Patron of Epileptics'; the monastery named for him in Alsace was a site of pilgrimage for those seeking a cure, and a hospital for epileptics was built there at the end of the fifteenth century. Quite a few other medieval saints were also patrons of epilepsy, including St Bibiana. A monastery named after her in Rome exported to Europe a powdered herb, hulwort, which was claimed to be a powerful epileptic cure if consumed in conjunction with a ceremonial three-Mass celebration.

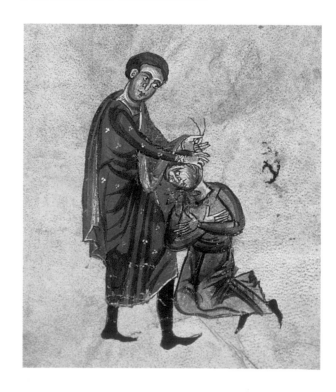

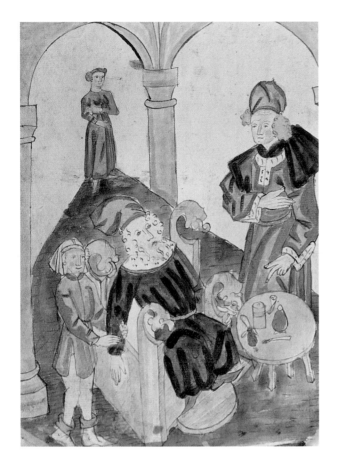

Not until the sixteenth century was the belief that epilepsy was physically contagious completely dispelled from medical thought. During the Renaissance, the medieval outlook was replaced by a more scientific attitude, and great strides were made in anatomical and clinical knowledge. The sixteenth-century physician Paracelsus wrote about epilepsy from both the pathological and psychiatric points of view. But, in general, theories of epilepsy advanced slowly. At the end of the sixteenth century the medical and superstitious views of epilepsy were in open conflict, supporters of both sides existing even within the medical profession itself, with those on the superstitious side invoking witchcraft and the devil as causes of the disease and magic as the appropriate treatment.

In the seventeenth and eighteenth centuries physicians had new tools in their exploration of the mysteries of epilepsy, for this was the period when modern chemistry and physics began to take shape. Many theories, both plausible and otherwise, attributed epilepsy to various chemical causes. It also became clear, through advances in anatomical knowledge, that the disease somehow emanated from the brain and that the nervous system had something to do with muscular convulsions. At the same time, religious excesses such as the Salem witch trials in America and the development of 'convulsionist' cults in Europe finally brought the debate over the natural or supernatural origins of epilepsy to a head. With the coming of the Enlightenment, the superstitious position was thoroughly

debunked by being stood on its head – the truth about medieval, ancient and even biblical stories of demoniacally possessed people was simply this: these people had merely been ill, they had been assumed to be possessed by others who knew no better, and such possession did not exist.

By the end of the eighteenth century, mental illness was at last becoming an interest of the medical profession, and insane asylums were becoming more like hospitals than prisons. Some epileptics were confined in such institutions, although they were not as closely restricted as the insane. (In Paris, the epileptics were let out on Sundays to attend Mass.) From the turn of the nineteenth century, there were scattered calls for separation of the two groups. One point of view was that epilepsy was contagious – not physically, as had previously been believed, but perhaps psychologically. It was feared that observing a seizure might, through imagination and sympathy, touch off a similar attack in the spectator, who could then develop the condition. Epileptics, then, were to be segregated not for their own protection, but to protect their insane, impressionable fellow-inmates.

But whether for the right or the wrong reasons, such segregation became a reality during the first half of the nineteenth century. In 1838 epileptic children in Paris were removed from the Hospital of the Incurably Ill to another location and even given some degree of education. By 1850 it was standard practice in Europe to house epileptics in segregated wards of insane asylums or large hospitals. Institutions specifically for epileptics came next, mostly created

A doctor visits his patient, from Treatise on Medicine, *fifteenth century, French Civic Museum, Colmar, France.*

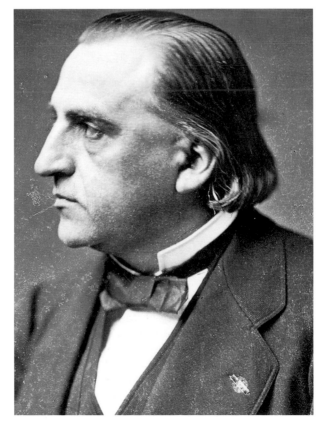

French physician Jean-Martin Charcot (1825–93) contributed much to knowledge of epilepsy and other neurological diseases, establishing a speciality in this field. One of his pupils was future psycho-analyst Sigmund Freud.

over the following fifty years. The result of segregation was that epilepsy began for the first time to receive specialized medical attention, mostly from physicians who worked in specialty hospitals or asylums. The psychiatric aspect of the disease started to attract some interest, and statistical thinking came into greater play.

Nonetheless, epilepsy research progressed slowly and fitfully over the first two-thirds of the nineteenth century. Success awaited developments in other areas of medicine, especially a more thorough understanding of the physiological functions of the brain and nervous system. A number of researchers during this period contributed to the foundations of what would become the field of neurology, among them the British physician John Hughlings Jackson, who had also spent many years making a special study of epilepsy.

Around 1880 Jackson, correlating and synthesizing the work of many of his colleagues, formulated a neurological theory of epilepsy involving multiple levels of sensory and motor functions of the nervous system, all governed by discharges from nerve cells ('neurons' – also the same as brain cells). Combined with the observations of French neurologist Jean-Martin Charcot, who distinguished 'hysteria' from epilepsy based on the physiological–neurological causes of the latter, Jackson's theory formed the basis for our understanding of epilepsy today.

Jackson's theory implied that the point of origin of the discharge causing a convulsion could be localized and treated, and soon British surgeons Victor Horsley and William MacEwan proved Jackson's ideas in practice. In 1886 Horsley reported three cases of epilepsy – two caused by head injuries and one by a tumor – that he had cured through successful brain surgery. In 1888 MacEwan reported the successful diagnosis of the location in the brain of a convulsive discharge, which had been achieved by observing the physical symptoms of the seizure.

The twentieth century has seen further progress, especially in treatment, although modern medical science has yet to map the full etiology of epilepsy. More and more researchers have come to believe that the condition should be termed a group of related illnesses rather than a single disease entity – 'the epilepsies' instead of just 'epilepsy'. Its multiplicity of causes and its complex and widely varying symptoms lend credence to this view.

Nowadays in the United States the disease seems most prevalent in infants and very young children, with birth defects and oxygen starvation among the identified causes. Another high-incidence group consists of people living in the decaying slums of some urban areas. Lead poisoning and drug addiction are suspected of being leading causes of epilepsy in these modern ghettoes. In other sections of the population epilepsy may be caused by brain damage from encephalitis or meningitis infections, or by head injuries, brain tumors or strokes. Genetic inheritance of the condition, although certainly a factor, is now thought to be less significant in causing epilepsy than was formerly believed. Nevertheless, people from families with a history of the disease are more likely than others to suffer abnormal brain discharges and seizures.

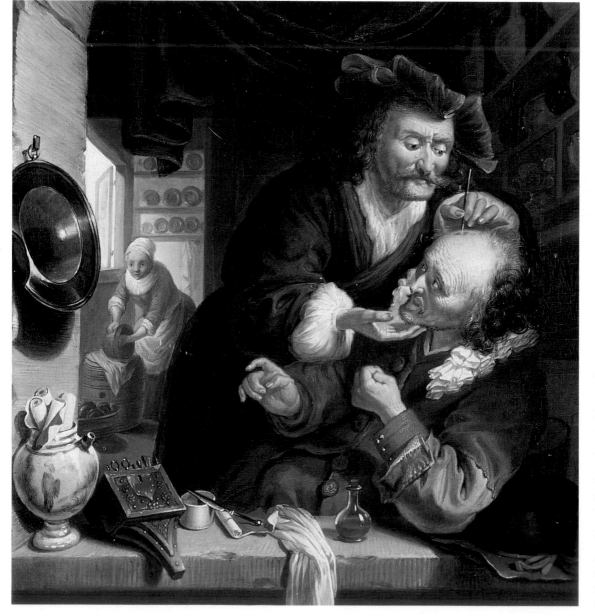

'The Barber Surgeon', by Koedyck (Koedijck) Isaac (c. 1616/18–68).

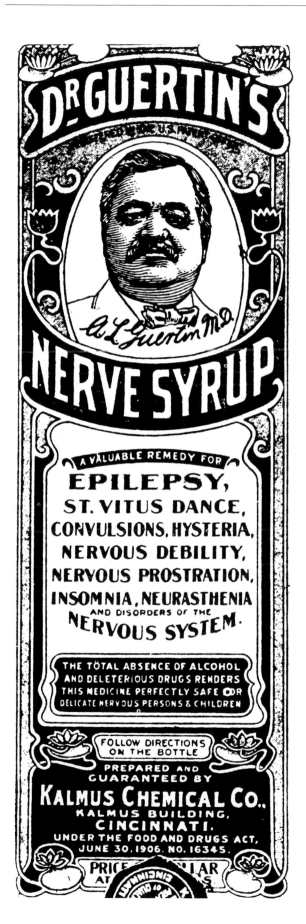

It is understood even better than in former times that not all seizures are evidence of epilepsy; non-epileptics and even epileptics themselves may experience 'pseudo-seizures', attacks that may look like epileptic seizures but which do not arise from the same causes. But pseudo-seizures, whether observed in an epileptic or a non-epileptic person, are extremely difficult to identify. Moreover, a known epileptic's seizures may be set off by virtually anything. A number of common triggers have been identified – for example, a separate illness, or overindulgence in alcohol – and it seems likely that stress is an underlying factor in many of them.

In recent times the use of the electroencephalograph has enabled medical researchers to monitor abnormal brain waves in epileptics and to some extent plot their locations. Seizures are now characterized by whether their brain activity is 'generalized' (meaning that abnormal discharges occur throughout the brain) or 'partial' (in which the discharges occupy only a portion of the brain). Partial seizures may produce widely varying symptoms – depending on what part of the brain is involved – and may pose formidable problems in diagnosis, whereas generalized seizures tend to affect much of the body as well as the brain and usually produce unconsciousness. A number of specific sub-types of seizure have been classified under the two overarching categories of generalized and partial. In addition, a 'secondarily generalized partial seizure', which begins in one part of the brain but then spreads throughout it, has been identified.

Nowadays seizures are usually controlled by medication. Perhaps 80 percent of all epileptics achieve full control over their seizures, but about one-third suffer side effects from the medication. In some cases, as in the 1880s, brain surgery may be a feasible alternative, especially if medication is unavailing, but usually only if the location of the epileptic discharges can be pinpointed.

Epilepsy is still seen throughout the world today and, like other diseases, is more likely to occur in places where people are poor, malnourished, and suffer the deleterious effects of overpopulation and inadequate medical care. As in the past, epileptics are generally misunderstood, feared and avoided. Only at the end of the twentieth century, and then only in the most 'advanced' nations, has there been any sign of a waning of the stigmatizing that epileptics have traditionally experienced.

Advertisment for Dr Guertin's Nerve Syrup – a popular specific, claiming to cure a wide range of diseases that were believed to be of the nervous system.

BIBLIOGRAPHY

Hirsch, August. 1883–6. *Handbook of Geographical and Historical Pathology* (trans. Charles Creighton), 3 vols. London.

Levy, Jerrold E. 1993. 'Epilepsy', in Kenneth F. Kiple (ed.), *The Cambridge World History of Human Disease*. Cambridge, England and New York.

Scott, Donald F. 1969. *About Epilepsy*. New York.

Temkin, Oswei. 1971. *The Falling Sickness: A History of Epilepsy from the Greeks to the Beginnings of Modern Neurology* (2nd edn, rev.). Baltimore.

The adjective 'scrofulous', from the Latin *scròfa*, originally meant something sow-like. By the Middle Ages scrofula (or scrophula) was employed to connote a vaguely defined disease-state of humans, a prominent symptom of which was swollen glands. In the nineteenth century the German epidemiologist August Hirsch explained that physicians of the past had used the word scrofula (or scrophula) to denote an 'inflammatory kind of tumor', especially when it appeared in the neck, but also in other parts of the body where lymph glands are located. Hirsch employed the term, yet it was becoming a nosological antique even as he penned it because of increasingly strident demands for a new precision from physicians determined to transform medicine from an art to a science. There was also another good reason for abandoning the use of the word. It carried connotations that were positively embarrassing to the *illuminati* still warming themselves in the sun of the Enlightenment.

For the German pioneer bacteriologist Robert Koch, whose claim in 1882 – correct, as it turned out, but skeptically reported by Hirsch – was to have found 'tubercle bacilli' in scrofulous glands, the disease was tuberculosis. But for Scottish physician William Cullen (1710–90), a man with a passion for classifying diseases, there were different kinds of scrofula. One was 'scrofula vulgaris' which was conceived of as the external form of the disease – an itch and rash developed in hospitals (probably the work of streptococci). The second was 'scrofula mesenterica' – the internal form of the illness – featuring symptoms of a swollen abdomen, appetite loss and pale countenance. Cullen's third kind, 'scrofula fugax' – neck swellings were its major symptom – was the type that Hirsch identified as scrofula a century later. The fourth kind was 'scrofula americana', that appeared among African slaves.

Prior to Cullen – and also to some extent contemporaneous with him – was another view of scrofula that had been prevalent especially in England and France since the middle of the thirteenth century. This was the conviction that, although scrofula was a real disease, it had a non-medical cure that was delivered by the touch of a king. In countries where people had faith in the touch the illness became known as the 'King's Evil' or the 'Royal Disease'.

Scrofula seems to have been mostly primary tuberculosis of the cervical lymph nodes. Before pasteurization, tuberculosis was frequently contracted when bacilli reached the body through the contaminated milk of tubercular cows. In addition tubercular mothers can pass the disease to unborn children. As a rule, however, the infection travels from human to human in airborne droplets expelled from infected persons.

Once inside the body, the bacilli find their way through the lymph channels to the closest lymph nodes. Thus, bacilli ingested in contaminated milk would tend to manifest their presence in the neck and intestinal regions, whereas those inhaled would concentrate in the lungs.

Because of this there is good reason to suspect that bovine tuberculosis, caused by drinking the milk of tubercular cows, was to blame for a large share of the tuberculosis cases called scrofula, or struma, meaning something built up. Clearly, Hirsch's survey points us in this direction. Europe, a large milk-drinking area, with its citizens also big consumers of other dairy products, was 'truly classic ground for scrofula'. Hirsch remarked that an 'untrustworthy' figure had about a quarter of the population of Great Britain suffering from the ailment. In fact, this may have been untrustworthy on the low side: others have reported that in the nineteenth century about half of the English population had the disease.

Predictably, Hirsch makes it clear that a large percentage of scrofula victims were children. Predictably for two reasons: the first is that the young have unusually low resistance to tuberculosis; and the second is that, as a rule, most adults residing in a place where tuberculosis was common would already have undergone their own bout with the primary infection during which the tubercle bacillus would have been eliminated. These would have been people with natural resistance sufficiently strong to triumph over the symptoms. In time the damaged patches in their organs would heal, and lymph glands return to normal size. Relatively few individuals infected by the tuberculosis bacilli go on to 'postprimary' infections (which in any event spread quite slowly) and develop the symptoms we have come to think of as typical. Moreover, bovine tuberculosis seldom progresses to pulmonary, and frequently lethal miliary tuberculosis. Scrofula, among the tubercular infections, seems seldom to have been fatal.

Very little of a biological nature was known about scrofula in the High Middle Ages. Although grounded in the theoretical and pragmatic knowledge of the ancients, medicine was a heady mixture that had also picked up elements of the supernatural, astrological, alchemical and even magical. Indeed, some physicians doubtless encouraged the notion that the touch of a king could cure this and perhaps other afflictions

CHAPTER 7

SCROFULA: THE KING'S EVIL AND STRUMA AFRICANA

By Kenneth F. Kiple

Little was known about scrofula in the Middle Ages. Physicians used the word to denote 'an inflammatory kind of tumor', especially in the neck. They believed a king's touch could cure it.

as well. Earlier monarchs had sometimes been credited with great healing powers, but the ritual of royal touching for scrofula seems to have begun with the kings of France after the return of Louis IX from the Crusades in 1254. Perhaps in the spirit of competition but probably also in an effort to find more favor with their subjects, their English counterparts, the Plantagenets, followed suit about a decade later.

Although we can only speculate about the reasons why the monarchs of England and France began the practice of touching for scrofula, we can be somewhat more certain why it was continued for the next half a millennium and longer. The symptoms of enlarged glands on the neck were highly visible to everyone – often they had become putrid. Visible as well were the frequently open sores on the neck and on the face. And, because most cases of primary tuberculosis resolve themselves in time, and such unsightly symptoms disappear, the king's touch must have seemed a truly miraculous cure to subjects and monarchs alike.

Touching could be hard work. On the basis of alms – 'the king's penny' – given for the touch, it has been calculated that in three different years England's Edward I (1272–1307) touched respectively 983, 1,219 and 1,736 scrofulous subjects. Some four and a half centuries later, Louis XV of France must have set an all-time record by touching more than 2,000 scrofula sufferers at his coronation in 1722.

The political benefits of such efforts could be enormous. In England, the last Anglo-Saxon King, Edward (1003–66)

known as the 'Confessor' because of his piety, was credited with great healing powers thought to stem from his holiness. He was proclaimed a saint in 1161 and, by taking up Edward the Confessor's healing tradition, the Plantagenets were, in effect, linking themselves with saintliness.

In the seventeenth and eighteenth centuries the political advantages of touching became even more pronounced, as the touch became a foundation for the claim of kings to rule by divine right. If the power of the royal touch to cure was given by God only to a true line of kings, then the act of curing was proof of belonging to a true line. As a consequence the touch was used to legitimate claims to thrones and the occupation of them.

In France and pre-Reformation England the religious nature of the touching ceremony also helped to keep relations harmonious between altar and throne and to maintain their mutual support. With the Reformation, however, Protestants began increasingly to find the ceremony too pagan for their taste and, by the time of the Stuart kings, they found it downright threatening. This was especially true during the reign of Charles I (1600–49) because of his insistence that kings had the 'divine right' to do what they pleased. An archenemy of the Puritans, Charles, like his father James I, was a champion of the theory of the 'divine right of kings', and, like his father, used the touch to justify his rule as a direct representative of God. As an upholder of the Church of England, a staunch opponent of Puritanism and an autocrat, Charles eventually lost his head to

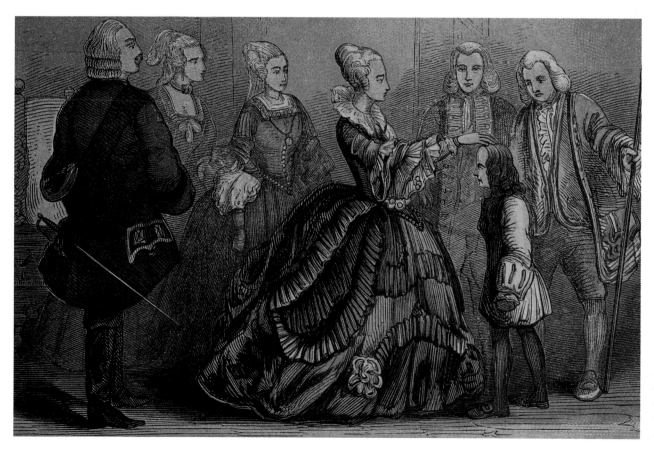

Queen Anne, the last of the Stuarts to touch for scrofula, touches Dr Samuel Johnson when he was a boy, to cure him of scrofula, or 'king's evil'.

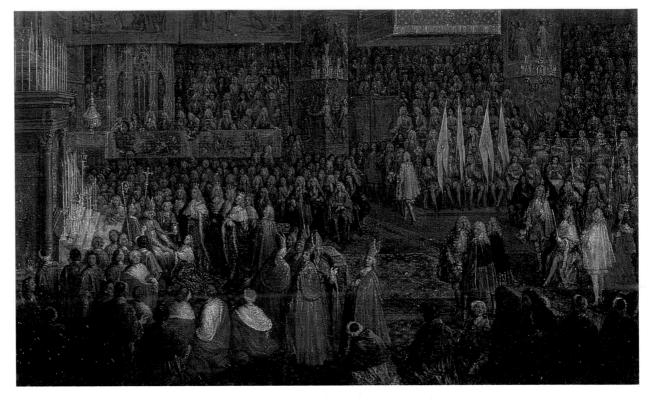

Coronation of Louis XV, 25 October 1722. Painting by Jean-Baptiste Martin (1659–1735). Chateau de Versailles, France.

the forces of Parliament and Puritanism, but the touch was continued by the Stuarts in exile.

It is difficult to imagine the crowds pressing in on the Stuart kings – the thousands upon thousands who came hoping for a cure or just to watch miracles in the making. The Puritans and Parliamentarians understood political danger when they saw it,

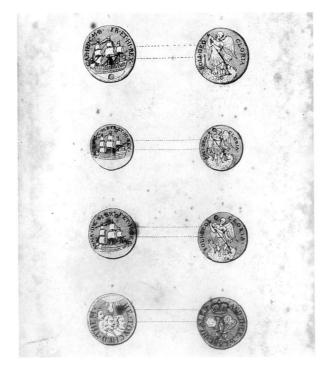

An etching of the two sides of four coin-like tokens known as 'Royal touch pieces' given to sufferers of the 'King's evil' by the King or Queen who touched them.

and they certainly saw it in this bond between the Stuarts and their subjects. But severing the head of a king had not severed the bond because the vast majority of Englishmen were hostile to the ideals that had inspired the armies of Cromwell, and with the fall of the Protectorate and the restoration of Charles II in 1660, the touch was resumed.

For Richard Wiseman, physician to Charles II and a rabid royalist, the Restoration seemed nothing less than an expression of the will of God that had returned the real line of kings to the throne. He urged using the touch to show that the king could cure where medicine could not, personally selected the most difficult cases to be sent to the king, and even wrote a book on scrofula and its royal cure. Perhaps as a result, in 1684 the largest ever number of applicants for the touch was recorded, and many were trampled to death in attempting to reach the hand of the king.

During the rule of the Catholic James II, which began in 1685, the touch doubtless played a role in the resurrection of the Stuarts' insistence on their divine rights. James, however, was scarcely comfortable on the throne when he was driven from it in 1688, and by the time of the last of the Stuarts to use the touch (and to sit on the throne of England, for that matter), much had changed. Anne, who became Queen Anne of England in 1702, was a staunch Protestant, Parliament was sovereign, and the divine right of kings was no longer an issue. Anne, nonetheless, felt compelled to continue the Stuart tradition of the touch. According to his biographer, Samuel Johnson was touched (but not cured) by the queen in 1712.

When the Hanoverian line of succession followed the Stuarts, there was no longer any political advantage to be gained by using the touch; in fact, quite the contrary, because Whig supporters scorned the ritual as medieval and superstitious.

The practice continued, however, in France until 1789 and there was one more brief, but failing, effort to revive it after the restoration of the Bourbons to buttress Charles X (1824–30) on the throne.

In a nineteenth century which had abandoned the belief that 'true' kings ruled by divine right, there was no longer any 'King's Evil'. Cynically, it seemed that scrofula was regarded as the King's Evil, curable by the touch of a monarch, only when and where it was politically advantageous. In Germany, Italy and other countries in Europe with no doctrine of a true line of kings, scrofula was seldom even viewed as a disease; rather its various symptoms were seen as manifestations of different diseases.

But quite apart from the decline in importance of the divine right issue there was another very good reason for the disappearance of the touch. By the time the eighteenth century had gotten underway, the medieval world view that had accepted the ability of monarchs to cure with a touch was rapidly disappearing. Although the common people only reluctantly abandoned their belief in such miracles, the educated classes had come to regard the touch as a useless superstition. This was, after all, the Age of the Enlightenment, and some of the medical books of the era reveal an enlightened embarrassment that there had ever been a time when people could have conceived of such silliness – a disease with a non-medical cure indeed! Throughout the century, rational skepticism continued to erode faith in any royal power to heal, so that in the nineteenth century Hirsch could write thirty-seven pages on scrofula and never once mention the phenomenon of the touch.

Meanwhile, across the Atlantic a disease called 'scrofula' had captured the attention of physicians, especially in the southern United States and in the West Indies. There scrofula – often called struma africana – was reputed to be rife among the slaves, and was thought of as a 'negro disease'.

Some planters blamed the condition on poor diets given to slaves by others less generous than themselves. There was also the suspicion that the slaves' habit of covering their heads with blankets while sleeping was to blame. Whatever the cause, the disease was viewed as lethal. A Kentucky physician wrote that scrofula was the 'great Scourge of Negroes'. He preferred to call it struma africana; others seized upon appellations such as 'cachexia africana', Negro poison and Negro consumption. Names such as scrofula, struma and consumption hint that physicians thought they were dealing with a tubercular condition. The lymphatic swellings in the neck and abdomen were hardly rare among whites in the United States and autopsies on black scrofula victims had

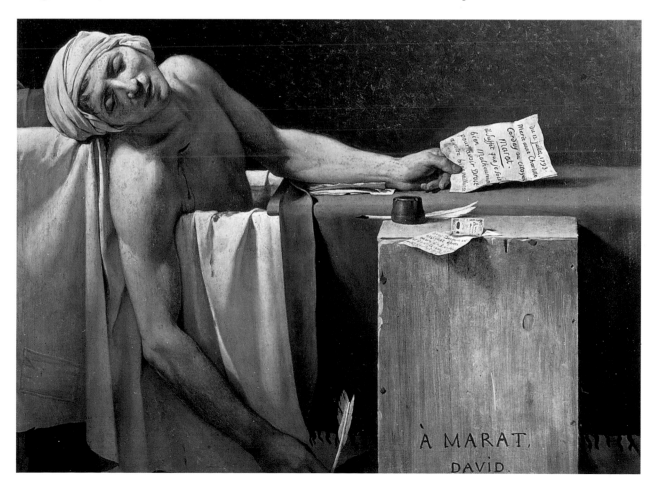

'The Death of Marat', 1793, by Jacques Louis David (1748–1825). Marat, killed in his bath by Charlotte Corday, found bathing relieved his many skin complaints.

revealed organs 'studded with tubercles'. Yet physicians stubbornly clung to the conviction that scrofula, with its enlarged cervical glands, was exclusively a 'negro' disease, born of a 'negro' constitution, and not 'consumption' (another term for tuberculosis) as they understood it.

They were right in that the disease could not have been bovine tuberculosis as was probably most frequently the case when whites in the United States, as in Europe, developed scrofula. The slaves had mostly originated from Africa's tropical regions, where tsetse flies made the raising of cattle and other large animals impossible. This meant that they did not have a history of milk-drinking and, consequently, were almost uniformly lactose intolerant – meaning that they could not digest the lactose in milk. Equally important, the slaves had been transported from one non-dairying region in the Old World to another in the New World. In the slave economies there was little or no access to milk or milk products by either blacks or whites.

Cartoon (1848) of 'The Sweating Cure', alleged to relieve a variety of skin diseases.

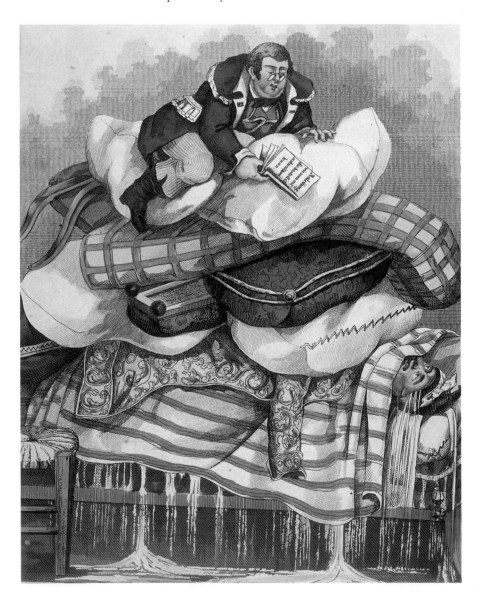

The ecological circumstances of the Africans' homelands, however, may hold more significance in resolving the problem of the identity of struma africana than merely the genetics of lactose intolerance. This is because Africans with roots south of the Sahara were familiar with, and therefore had developed some resistance to, most Eurasian diseases. Smallpox, measles, diphtheria and a host of other plagues had reached out to them over the millennia from beyond the desert and across the Indian Ocean. But tuberculosis was not one of these diseases. It was brought late to Africa by the Europeans and, consequently, both Africans at home and those transported abroad were virgin soil people for this particular pestilence.

From the experience of other populations facing tuberculosis for the first time, we know a great deal about what such a vulnerable state can mean. Native Americans, for example, who were unaware of the disease until the Europeans introduced it, have provided us with a dreadful lesson, as tuberculosis gradually became their biggest killer. The slowness of its spread was such, however, that the malady reached a remote tribe in Western Canada only at the beginning of the twentieth century. Terrible as their subsequently drawn-out struggle with the disease proved to be – and one which physicians could only watch helplessly – it did have the heuristic effect of providing a crystal-clear picture of tuberculosis loose among persons with little immunological ability to resist it.

Most germane for that picture is that the first and second generations of Indians to be stricken manifested few pulmonary symptoms which physicians were trained to recognize. Rather, patients revealed extensive glandular involvement, and the only reason the physicians knew that they were dealing with tuberculosis was because their microscopes told them so. It was only with the third generation under assault that the disease began to show a predilection for settling in the lungs, and glandular involvement had fallen to 7 percent of cases. With the fourth generation, only 1 percent of cases had glandular symptoms.

What observers were witnessing was the ability of the human body to adapt to tuberculosis. In the inexperienced bodies of first and second generations of Indians the bacilli of tuberculosis met with such sluggish and ineffective resistance that the disease was able to race through lymph channels and spread to numerous organs. But the bodies of third and especially fourth generations were learning to cope with the disease – most effectively accomplished by walling it up in the lungs. In addition, those most susceptible to the illness were brutally weeded out: initially the disease generated an incredible annual mortality rate of about 9 percent of the population.

It is instructive to apply the lessons from this example to the earlier phenomenon of scrofula among the slaves. Their bodies, too, were inexperienced with tuberculosis. Although the disease was carried to Africa by the Europeans, they seldom penetrated inland during the days of the slave trade. Consequently, it seems reasonable to assume that the disease spread very slowly south of the Sahara – so slowly, in fact, that the overwhelming majority of Africans forced into the slave trade had probably never been in contact with it.

Nor were they likely to encounter it in the enforced isolation of plantations in the American South or West Indies where they were quarantined, as it were, from those urban environments that bred tuberculosis. Hence when Antebellum physicians and their counterparts in the West Indies were faced with a disease among slaves which showed extensive glandular symptoms, they thought it a peculiarly negro kind of scrofula or struma africana.

If this hypothesis is to stand up, then we must have evidence that this unidentifiable tuberculosis did finally become recognizable as it did with the Western Canadian Indians. Unfortunately such evidence was forthcoming in terrible abundance. After slavery was abolished in the United States and the West Indies the disease burst upon the freed men as 'consumption' in a medically recognizable form and for a few decades generated some of the highest tuberculosis mortality rates in the world.

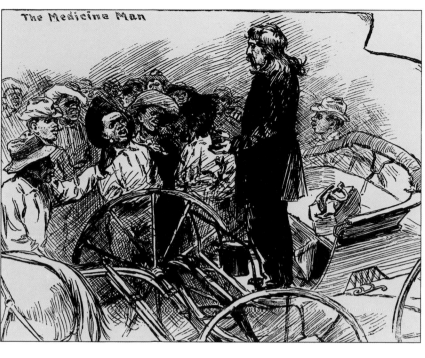

The Medicine Man

Pen-and-ink sketch of a 'medicine' man in the South selling panaceas to freed slaves from his one-horse shay in 1883.

BIBLIOGRAPHY

French, Roger K. 1993. 'Scrofula (Scrophula)', in Kenneth F. Kiple (ed.), *The Cambridge World History of Human Disease*. Cambridge, England and New York.

Hirsch, August. 1883–86. *Handbook of Historical and Geographical Pathology* (tr. Charles Creighton), 3 vols. London.

Johnston, William D. 1993. 'Tuberculosis', in Kenneth F. Kiple (ed.), *The Cambridge World History of Human Disease*. Cambridge, England and New York.

Kiple, Kenneth F. 1884. *The Caribbean Slave: A Biological History*. Cambridge, England and New York.

Dubos, René and Jean. 1952. *The White Plague* (1987 edn). New Brunswick and London.

McGrew, Roderick E. 1985. *Encyclopedia of Medical History*. New York.

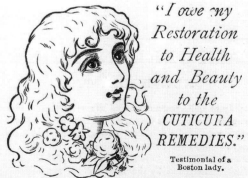

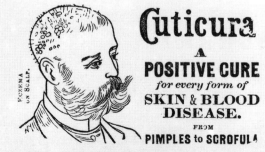

"*I owe my Restoration to Health and Beauty to the* CUTICURA REMEDIES."

Testimonial of a Boston lady.

DISFIGURING Humors, Humiliating Eruptions, Itching Tortures, Scrofula, Salt Rheum and Infantile Humors cured by the CUTICURA REMEDIES.

CUTICURA RESOLVENT, the new blood purifier, cleanses the blood and perspiration of impurities and poisonous elements, and thus removes the *cause*.

CUTICURA, the great Skin Cure, instantly allays Itching and Inflammation, clears the Skin and Scalp, heals Ulcers and Sores, and restores the Hair.

CUTICURA SOAP, an exquisite Skin Beautifier and Toilet Requisite, prepared from CUTICURA, is indispensable in treating Skin Diseases, Baby Humors, Skin Blemishes, Chapped and Oily Skin.

CUTICURA REMEDIES are absolutely pure, and the only infallible Blood Purifiers and Skin Beautifiers.

Sold everywhere. Price, Cuticura, 50 cents; Soap, 25 cents; Resolvent, $1. POTTER DRUG AND CHEMICAL CO., BOSTON, MASS.

Cuticura A POSITIVE CURE *for every form of* SKIN & BLOOD DISEASE. FROM PIMPLES to SCROFULA

ITCHING, Scaly, Pimply, Scrofulous, Inherited, Contagious, and Copper Colored Diseases of the Blood, Skin and Scalp, with Loss of Hair, are positively cured by the CUTICURA REMEDIES.

CUTICURA RESOLVENT, the new blood purifier, cleanses the blood and perspiration of impurities and poisonous elements, and removes the cause.

CUTICURA, the great Skin Cure, instantly allays Itching and Inflammation, clears the Skin and Scalp, heals Ulcers and Sores, and restores the Hair.

CUTICURA SOAP, an exquisite Skin Beautifier and Toilet Requisite, prepared from CUTICURA, is indispensable in treating Skin Diseases, Baby Humors, Skin Blemishes, Chapped and Oily Skin.

CUTICURA REMEDIES are absolutely pure and the only infallible Blood Purifiers and Skin Beautifiers.

Sold everywhere. Price, Cuticura, 50 cents; Soap, 25 cents; Resolvent, $1. Prepared by POTTER DRUG AND CHEMICAL CO., BOSTON, MASS.

☞ Send for "How to Cure Skin Diseases."

Contemporary advertisements claiming to cure a wide range of skin complaints, including scrofula.

There are two diseases called leprosy. One produces lepers – the archetypical outcasts from society. The other, far simpler to explain, is a disease caused by infection with *Mycobacterium leprae*, and is sometimes known as 'Hansen's disease'.

The need to exclude or shun individuals from a community, to define the 'other', the outsider, seems to be fundamental to human societies. It is in the Old Testament that we first find this instinctive group behavior in connection with a word which is now translated as leprosy. In Leviticus, a book of codes and laws said to date to around 1000 BC, *tsara'ath* describes those who must be expelled to live 'without the camp'. Passages from Leviticus focus on the uncleanness of the leper himself, and on his path to healing in purgations and ritually determined periods of isolation; they describe his covering of his upper lip and croaking of the words 'Unclean, unclean!' Typically the priest had a part in making the diagnosis, and in restoring order and health to the body of the community by expelling the leper and ritually cleansing his dwelling.

The problem with biblical leprosy has always been that it does not much resemble any known infectious disease. The biblical description makes leprosy a disease of one's house:

'The Lord said to Moses and Aaron … when I put a leprous disease in a house in the land of your possession, then he who owns the house shall come and tell the priest, "There seems to be some sort of disease in my house." Then the priest shall command that they empty the house before the priest goes to examine the disease, lest all that is in the house be declared unclean; and afterward the priest shall go in to see the house. And he shall examine the disease; and if the disease is in the walls of the house with greenish or reddish spots, and if it appears to be deeper than the surface, then the priest shall go out of the house to the door of the house, and shut up the house seven days.'(Leviticus 14: 33–8)

Bacterial leprosy, Hansen's disease, is not what is described in the Leviticus text, however. Bacterial leprosy can cause considerable destruction of the upper lip and nose, and the bacteria often invade the nerves to the larynx and vocal cords, resulting in a harsh, rasping voice. The disease frequently causes patches of skin to lose their sensitivity to touch or pain, and in darker-skinned individuals such as the ancient Semites, the affected skin would be lighter, discolored, rough or in some other way distinctive. Nevertheless, it requires a great leap of imagination, together with a very selective reading of Leviticus, to connect the ritualized leprosy of the Old Testament with bacterial leprosy.

The Leviticus leprosy seems to be closer to the scaly, flaking, whitish skin affliction described in Greek Hippocratic writings as *lépra*. (Hence the familiar translation.) Both *lépra* and *tsara'ath* were considered curable. The Greco-Roman 'elephantiasis', still uncommon in Galen's day (*c.* 150–200 AD) has a much greater resemblance to bacterial infection with *Mycobacterium leprae*. The early stages of this affliction were called 'leontiasis', and bore many of the hallmarks of bacterial leprosy: a bad odor (related to multiple secondary infections), collapsed but flushed cheeks, thickened lips, swollen eyebrows. Popular tradition ascribed increased libidinal energies to these sufferers and so 'satyriasis' also became associated with elephantiasis. At the time of Celsus, Rufus of Ephesus, Pliny the Elder and even Galen, elephantiasis was seen as relatively new to the Empire and difficult to cure, the early symptoms being livid or black patches that became hideously ulcerated and were nearly impossible to heal. The word applied to this disease would also be translated as leprosy later on.

One of the great ironies of the twinned history of leprosy is that the bacterial infection from a tuberculosis-like microorganism may have first spread through the western Mediterranean at the same time as Christianity, with its Judaic textual tradition. Ancient non-Christian physicians and Roman encyclopedists traced the origins of the 'new'

CHAPTER 8

LEPROSY: LARGER THAN LIFE

By Ann G. Carmichael

In this medieval miniature a leper comes begging for alms, carrying his clapper and his bowl.

disease to Egypt, though they were not even sure that it was possible for a new disease to occur. At the same time the popular stigmatizing of *tsara'ath* increased, and the practice of excluding the afflicted individuals from the community echoed Rome's strategies for containing and consolidating its Empire against the barbarians.

There is no firm evidence that *M. leprae* did in fact evolve in Egypt, nor that it had any earlier home outside Europe and the Middle East. In early Vedic texts there are clinical descriptions of an 'ashen' disease, *kilasa*, with white, discolored skin patches and flaking, but it is probable that the disease was actually psoriasis rather than bacterial leprosy. However, Indian texts dating from the same period as the Greco-Roman ones mentioned above, refer to a great *kustha* disease, contagious by sex, touch and respiration, incurable, and having much the same progression of symptoms as elephantiasis.

Mirko Grmek has studied the behavior of Mycobacteriacea, a family that includes human and animal tuberculoses, and avian tuberculosis or 'scrofula'. *Mycobacterium leprae*, causing leprosy, is distinctive among the Mycobacteriacea because it only infects humans. In fact, one of the impediments to laboratory and clinical study of leprosy in the twentieth century was the difficulty in finding a susceptible animal host for experimentation. Individuals who have been exposed to

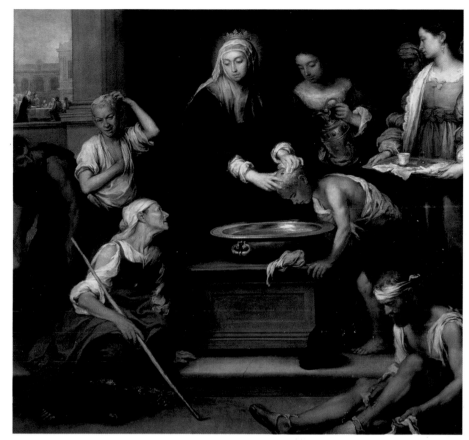

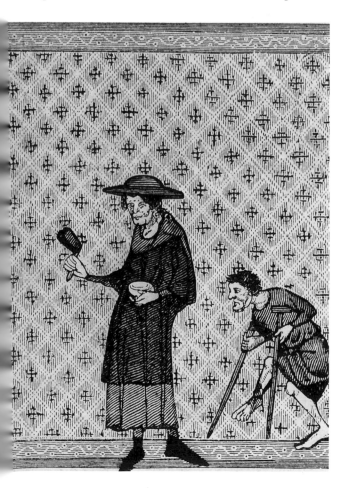

tuberculosis seem to be highly resistant to subsequent infection with leprosy, although the reverse is not true. To Grmek the ancient evidence suggested that *M. leprae* probably evolved from other mycobacteria, and that it was a by-product of urbanization.

As the Church tried to spread the message of Christianity in medieval Europe, biblical leprosy seemed to provide a powerful connection between sin and disease, reinforcing the role of the clergy in humankind's salvation. Thus, in the Middle Ages, the disease was deliberately linked to biblical accounts of leprosy and methods for controlling it.

As well as the Leviticus references, there are other mentions of leprosy: stories of redemption and punishment, of God's mercy as well as His judgment. Lazarus, in the New Testament, described as 'sick and disabled', tried to acquire some of Christ's power of physical healing by touching Him. The story was an elegantly simple metaphor for conveying the message of spiritual healing that the Church and the clergy offered. In the earlier Middle Ages the clergy were among the few educated men with access to ancient medical texts. Moreover, the churches, shrines and monasteries of that period were often built on or near pre-Christian healing and holy sites, in order to reinforce the messages of healing and salvation.

Another biblical leper was Job. Once a good and religious man, Job was tested by God: he was stripped of his belongings and friends, and then stricken with hideous sores. Disease and suffering are depicted as a form of martyrdom

St Elizabeth of Hungary tending the sick and leprous, by Bartoleme Esteban Murillo (1617–82). Hospital de la Santa Caridad, Seville.

and as a test of faith. But Job's case undermined the usual attribution of sickness to sin, and thus the justification for the exclusion of the leper.

During the early Middle Ages these tales were regarded as useful moral exemplars, even though they justified the Old Testament practice of excluding the lepers from society. The first Christian emperor, Constantine, although he ordered the expulsion of lepers, also observed the newer, Christian ideal of caring for the sick – a means of personal salvation – by assigning a minister to serve the outcasts.

In the twelfth century the number of hospice institutions devoted to caring for the occasional leper increased exponentially. Suddenly leprosaria, specialized asylums for lepers, appeared throughout western Europe. Laws relating to the diagnosis, control and care of lepers proliferated, while Church-generated texts describing the dangers to spiritual wellbeing and public health from lepers, echoed similar concerns about the presence of Jews and heretics.

By 1179, when Church authorities met at the Third Lateran Council dedicated to the reform of Christendom, attention was given to the problem of leprosy: lepers were to be identified and segregated. From the time of their separation they had to carry bells or clappers – usually straps of leather or slices of wood bound by iron so that they made a distinctive noise when waved – to make their presence known. They were required to wear a yellow cross on their garb, and in some places had to carry a long stick for reaching for goods or alms in public places. The world of the leper was outside the safety of walled cities and towns, a world belonging to bandits and other wild creatures. The banishment of the leper has survived in popular imagination, as in this evocative scene by Robert Louis Stevenson:

'Upon this path, stepping forth from the margin of the wood, a white figure now appeared. It paused a little and seemed to look about; and then, at a slow pace, and bent almost double, it began to draw near across the heath. At every step the bell clanked. Face, it had none; a white hood,

'Beggar Lazarus and the Rich Man's Table'. Panel by Kasper van der Hoecke (d. 1648). Lazarus, with his clapper, lies starving, while a dog licks his sores.

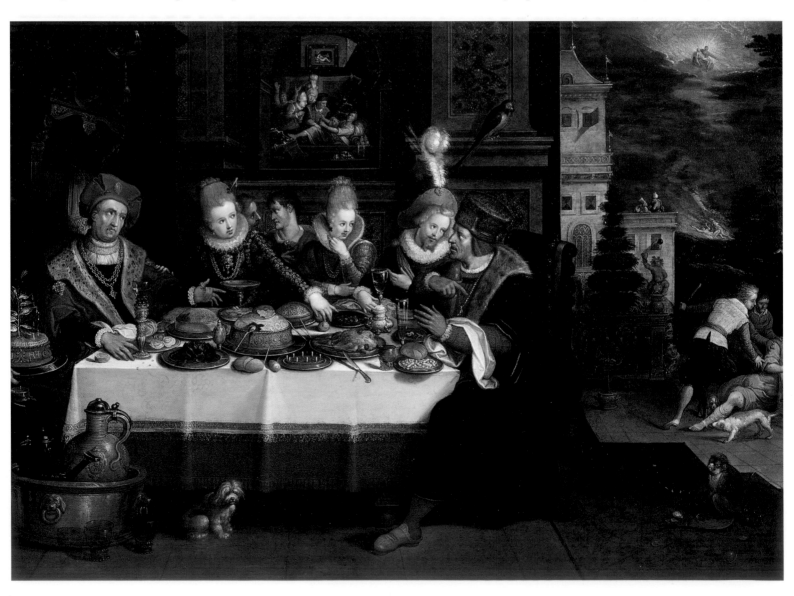

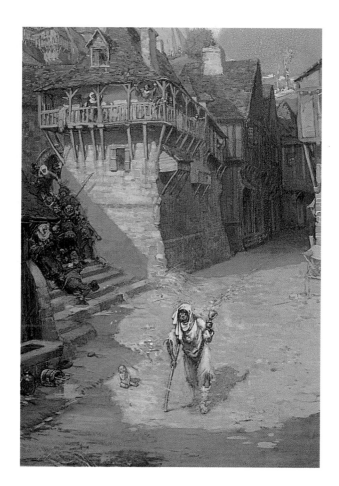

caused by repeated frostbite and subsequent gangrene. But the fusion of small bones of the hands and feet, so that the remains look like a bear's claw, and the 'pencilling' of the remaining digits, are fairly characteristic of advanced leprosy persuasive evidence that the bacterial disease existed in medieval Europe.

The second kind of evidence for medieval bacterial leprosy, less tangible to be sure, is even more convincing than the Roman descriptions of elephantiasis. Arabic-Persian medical texts, particularly the tenth-century *Canon of Medicine* by Avicenna, give descriptions of the distinctive changes to the face characteristic of leprosy: the loss of the eyebrows and eyelashes, the thickening of the skin across the nasal bridge and the loss of 'free play' of facial expression, as well as the hoarseness of the voice and the 'thickening' of the blood, seen when the blood of a putative leper is swirled in a wooden bowl.

As the works of Avicenna, with their diagnostic descriptions of leprosy, were translated into Latin and increasingly accepted by university physicians in the west, the apparent incidence of leprosy declined. After 1300, wherever the diagnosis of leprosy was entrusted to well-informed physicians rather than to churchmen or enthusiastic lay officials, the occurrences of the disease decreased.

Leprosy, both biblical and bacterial, apparently declined steadily through the later Middle Ages, for a number of reasons: better medical diagnostics; depopulation caused by the Black Death and recurrent bubonic plague; effective segregation of lepers from the general community; and

People scrambling to get away from a leper, who rings his bell to warn them. In this watercolour by R. Cooper, someone has carelessly left an infant on the leper's roadside path.

Purification of a knight from a fourteenth-century manuscript. Many believed that 'true' leprosy followed in the wake of the Crusades, the returning knights bringing the disease back with them.

not even pierced with eyeholes, veiled the head; and as the creature moved, it seemed to feel its way with the tapping of a stick. Fear fell upon the lads, as cold as death. "A leper!" said Dick, hoarsely. "His touch is death," said Matcham. "Let us run."'

It is only too easy to see the overwhelming attention devoted to the problem of leprosy in the High Middle Ages as a response to a real, rapidly spreading bacterial disease. Thus many have speculated that 'true' leprosy followed in the wake of the Crusades, the Europeans' first massive foray outside Europe. In this view, Crusaders returned horribly infected, their disease visible to all. It can also be argued that churchmen, intent on consolidating power and control, used leprosy as a way of justifying the need for new forms of public control.

Two different kinds of evidence from the 1200s and 1300s bear witness to the existence of *M. leprae* in Europe. In the 1950s the Danish paleopathologist Vilhelm Møller-Christensen and his associates examined skeletons found in graveyards attached to traditional leprosaria in Denmark, particularly in a leper community at Naestved. The corpses had been buried ritualistically, always with the head facing east, and the skeletons all bore evidence of infection consistent with *M. leprae*. Other disease processes might account for some of the deformities: for example, missing toes and fingers, and damage to the upper lip and nasal region could have been

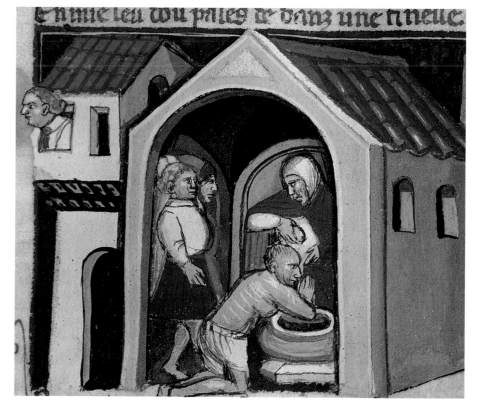

the rise of urbanization leading to increased prevalence of tuberculosis. Some older studies also speculate that leprosy was at first confused with syphilis, particularly because the medieval leper was depicted as extraordinarily lecherous. However, most of the proponents of this theory are principally interested in showing that syphilis was not first introduced to Europe around 1500. By the sixteenth century, the number of lepers in special hospitals

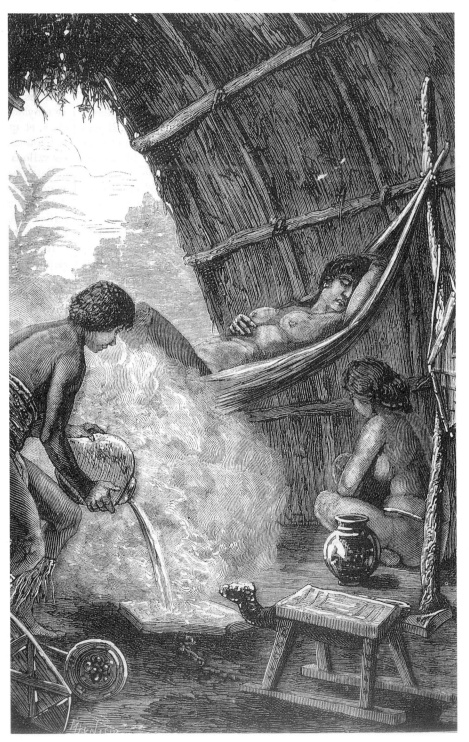

Steam bath cure for leprosy by South American natives, c. 1880.

was very low, and these hospitals were frequently seized for other purposes.

Europeans' interest in leprosy declined precipitately, however, until the middle years of the nineteenth century, when bacterial and biblical leprosy surged dramatically. Again the bacterial history is the simpler tale.

Norwegian physicians were becoming increasingly concerned with the health, working and living conditions of Norway's predominantly rural population. Enlightened clergy played an important role in focusing attention specifically on leprosy – for scabies, scurvy, worm infestations, tuberculosis, syphilis and even starvation were also widely prevalent.

In 1816 a pastor in Bergen offered a report to a medical journal, describing the destitute peasants seeking care at a nearby leprosarium, St Jørgens hospital, which had been established in the fifteenth century. This sparked off scientific interest and, in 1832, a survey of leprosy in Norway was undertaken with the aid of local parish ministers. Several censuses in the 1840s and 1850s pointed to a significant problem with this disease, highlighting the need to standardize diagnosis in 'modern' medical terms. Daniel Cornelius Danielssen, a physician at St Jørgens, and C. W. Boeck published a series of studies on the subject, providing the impetus for the creation of a national, government-sponsored leprosy research center in Bergen by 1849. Danielssen and Boeck published a survey of the disease in Europe, specifically linking it to the elephantiasis of Greco-Roman medical tradition.

Danielssen and Boek are also responsible for the clinical differentiation of two separate types of bacterial leprosy, still accepted today. One of these they called tubercular, because the victims bore nodular tubercles that would inevitably progress to destroy the facial features and usually caused blindness and severe deformities. Nowadays this form of bacterial leprosy is known as 'low resistant', meaning that the victim has little resistance to the replication of the bacteria, and so the disease is clinically more severe. It is also called 'leonine' leprosy, after the lion-like face it produces, a destructive process that had been described by Avicenna centuries earlier. The second type of leprosy Danielssen and Boeck called 'anesthetic', now known as 'high resistant'. (Confusingly, it was called 'tubercular' in the slightly older medical and historical literature.) This milder form of leprosy produces patchy areas of anesthesia on the skin, but often progresses quite slowly and can even be arrested with good nursing care and antibiotic therapy.

The Norwegian work on leprosy tried to dispel old myths: that leprosy was caused by eating spoiled fish, for example, or easily spread by airborne contagion. In fact, Danielssen and Boeck believed that leprosy was an inherited condition that could be readily distinguished from other skin afflictions.

On the one hand, the attention and resources devoted to Norwegian lepers led to their concentration in treatment centers, and to a kind of focused research that was possible nowhere else in Europe. It is little wonder that the discovery of the microorganism unique to bacterial leprosy was made in a Bergen hospital, by Gerhard Henrik Armauer Hansen in 1873. On the other hand, the theory that leprosy could be inherited was increasingly discredited among the researchers of the later nineteenth century, deflecting attention from the enlightened example Norway had set for the care of lepers.

An epidemic of leprosy in the Hawaiian islands in the 1860s once again revived interest in the disease. The epidemic was both dramatic and highly visible. A series of imported diseases had caused a devastating decline in the native population, and Asian laborers were imported in order to maintain colonial programs there. The leprosy epidemic coincided with the introduction of the Asian laborers and led to the revival of ideas about the treatment of lepers that Danielssen and Boeck had rejected: the isolation of all lepers and a racist view of the disease. Although over 90 percent of newly identified lepers were native Hawaiian, the epidemic was linked to Chinese immigration and the disease called 'true Oriental leprosy'.

In 1865 Hawaii's colonial government purchased land for the lepers on the volcanic island of Molokai, hemmed in on three sides by the sea, and on the fourth by a formidable mountain barrier.

Colonial governments generally did not accept an obligation to provide welfare relief to indigenous populations, and Hawaii's government, including its nascent Board of Health, was adamant in this respect. Instead, they emphasized the extreme contagiousness of the disease, and hence the necessity of protecting the healthy. In 1873, when Hansen was training his microscope on tissue taken from leprous nodules, a Belgian Catholic priest, Joseph Damien de Veuster, resolved to bring spiritual and medical care to the Hawaiians on Molokai, who had been left to care for themselves.

Armaeur Hansen. At the 1897 International Leprosy Conference in Berlin, Hansen finally received due acclaim for his work on the disease.

Trading between nations was a major contributory factor in the spread of contagious diseases, particularly leprosy.

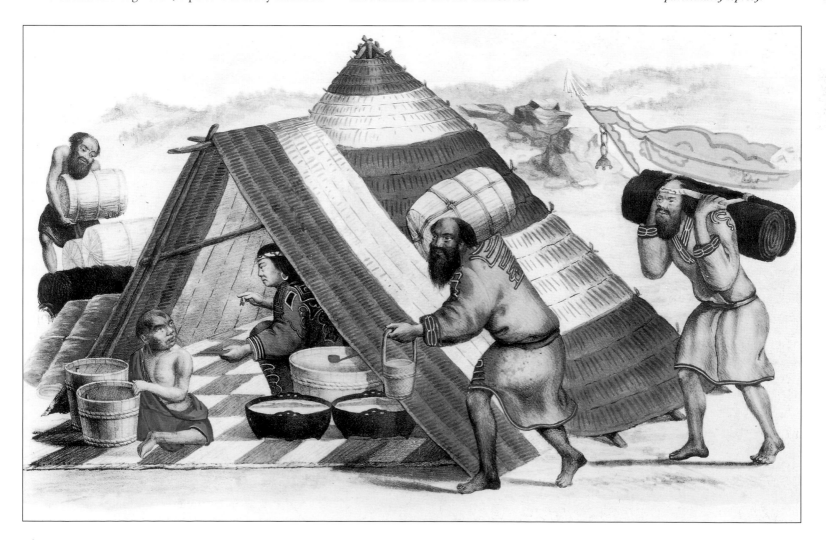

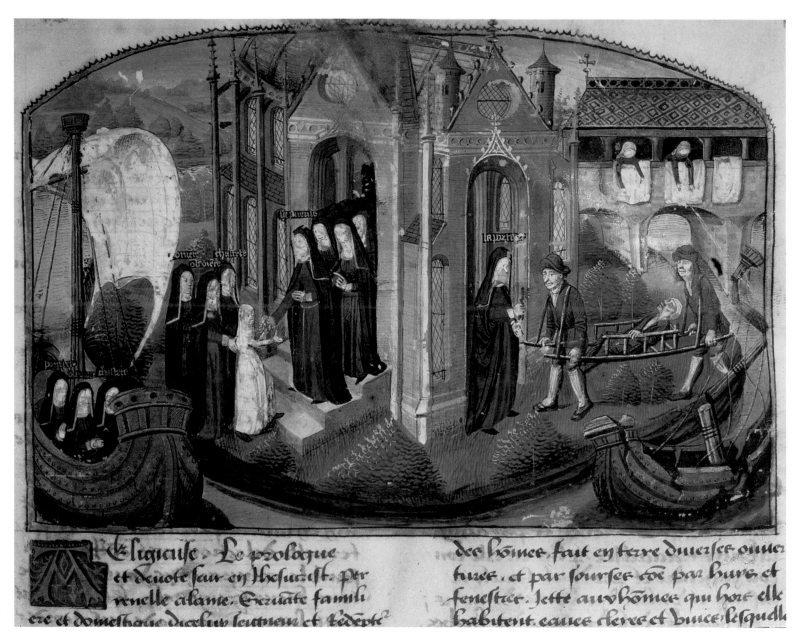

Eligieuse Le prologue
et deuote seur en Ihesucrist. per
renelle alame. Seruate famili
ere et domesthaie dicesur seruneu et tederte

dee hômes fait en terre duerses ouuer
tures. et par sourses et par hurs et
fenestres. Jette aux hômes qui hore elle
habitent. eaues cleres et biues lesquelh

'Nun entering the Hôtel de Dieu, admission of a sick man.' Book illustration from 1482/3, with depictions of life in the Hôtel de Dieu in Paris.

Missionary fervor, the dedicated exportation of the Christian message and texts, aided and abetted both the Hawaiian government's plan of action and Father Damien's intervention. Robert Louis Stevenson visited Molokai in 1889, and spent twelve days with the saintly, leprosy-ridden Father Damien. He expressed his sentiments in a poem:

'To see the infinite pity of this place,
The mangled limb, the devastated face,
The innocent sufferers smiling at the rod,
A fool were tempted to deny his God.'

Father Damien died soon afterwards. In the 1880s and 1890s leprosy, in both its bacterial and biblical presences, sprang to view as never before: concern focused on the primitiveness, the Asianness, the tropical otherness of the disease; it was seen as a distinct, immanent danger to the west if allowed to proceed uncontrolled. Despite clear and mounting epidemiological evidence that it posed no such threat, the exaggerated Biblical description of the contagiousness of leprosy evoked predict-able public responses and dictated extreme colonial inter-ventions. The Prince of Wales instituted a National Leprosy Fund in 1893, which sponsored a Leprosy Commission to investigate the disease in British India. The first international conference devoted to leprosy was held in Berlin in 1897, sponsored by the emperor of Germany. Just two years earlier Kaiser Wilhelm II had dubbed leprosy 'a yellow peril'. A cartoon of a Buddha astride a Chinese dragon emerging from the smoke of a burning Europe, was captioned: 'Nations of Europe! Join in Defense of Your Faith and Your Home!'

By the end of the nineteenth century the United States was engaged in war with Spain, and eagerly absorbed the scientific consensus that 'every leper is a danger to his surroundings'. When cases of leprosy were recognized among US veterans of the Philippines campaign, the American colonial government quickly created two large isolation facilities for patients in the islands of Cúlion and Cebu, and, a decade later, a leper asylum near Carville, Louisiana. American concern with leprosy and strict patient isolation lacked the strong missionary basis of European intervention in Asia, but nevertheless enthusiastically embraced the biblical mandate for seclusion and separation. Meanwhile, British campaigns in India resulted in the establishment of ninety-four leprosy asylums by 1921, most supported by Christian missions.

In retrospect, it is surprising that until quite recently treatment of lepers largely followed medieval practices, including the stigmatization of the leper, the segregation of the sexes and reliance on religious education rather than on scientific and clinical study. Leprosy was seen as far more attractive as a problem for philanthropy than for medicine.

BIBLIOGRAPHY

Brody, Saul N. 1974. *The Disease of the Soul: Leprosy in Medieval Literature*. Ithaca.

Grmek, Mirko D. 1989. *Diseases in the Ancient Greek World* (trans. M. and L. Muellner). Baltimore and London.

Gussow, Zachary. 1989. *Leprosy, Racism, and Public Health: Social Policy in Chronic Disease Control*. San Francisco and London.

Moore, R. I. 1987. *The Formation of a Persecuting Society: Power and Deviance in Western Europe*, pp. 950–1250. Oxford and Cambridge, Massachusetts.

Ober, William B. 1987. 'Can the leper change his spots? The iconography of leprosy', chapter 6 in *Bottoms Up! A Pathologist's Essays on Medicine and the Humanities*. Carbondale.

Stevenson, Robert Louis. 1925 [1884]. *The Black Arrow*. South Seas Edition of the collected works, vol. XVII. New York.

This turn-of-the-century leprosarium in Jerusalem shows all the obvious forms of leprosy: inmates with bandaged hands and feet, ravaged faces, and crutches, as well as the enduring presence of Christian charity.

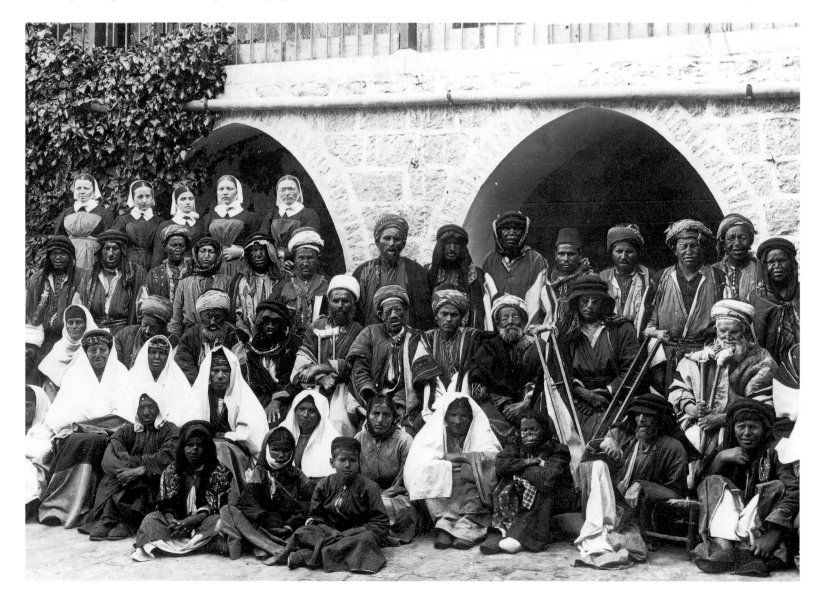

PURVEYORS OF PESTILENCE: URBANISM, WAR, TRADE AND IMPERIALISM

As a rule, the birth of cities was a messy business. They developed as open sewers into which rodents burrowed and above which swarms of insects hovered. The people who lived in them seldom washed, and their hair, skin, bowels and breath were alive with pathogens. In short, cities were magnets for myriad diseases and mortality was such that their populations had to be continually replenished with new arrivals from the countryside. But perhaps paradoxically cities also helped to tame many plagues by rendering them endemic. In epidemic form diseases such as measles or smallpox swept over populations killing or immunizing so many that they disappeared, only to reappear when another generation of non-immunes had arisen to be slaughtered. Yet gradually, painfully, cities became sufficiently populous that enough newborns were produced annually to retain diseases on a year-round basis. Epidemics that in the past had arrived periodically to assault people of all ages now became childhood ailments. And because most such illnesses treat children more gently than adults they immunized each generation against future attacks.

Troops on the march, such as those of the Turkish and Mongol conquerors between 1000 and 1500, or the Crusaders who tried to check them, spasmodically united the cities of the eastern and western realms of the known world and thus their pools of diseases. But it was trade that more steadily knitted them together, and it was a quest to revolutionize such trade that impelled the Portuguese down the African coast to tie this huge Old World appendage closer to its core. Less than a century later the Europeans, led by Spain and Portugal, embarked on a career of imperialism that progressively drew the other stray chunks of Pangaea (the Americas, Oceania, New Zealand and Australia) into their vortex as well. A long-term consequence of all of this was a homogenization of the planet's food supply that stimulated population growth on a global scale. But in the short term, the result was demographic disaster for practically all of the New World peoples suddenly face to face with Old World pathogens.

Although almost any disease discussed in this book could have been included under the 'urbanism, war, trade and imperialism' rubric, those that are focused on in this section are especially representative. In the case of urbanism, as was just noted, cities, although breeding grounds of disease, were also instrumental in reducing plagues such as measles or smallpox to childhood diseases. In the case of trade, after a hiatus of many centuries, bubonic plague once more reached Europe via trade with the East – this time across the caravan routes. Or to blame trade again, about half of the Portuguese *marinheiros* (seamen) who sailed with Vasco da Gama around the Cape of Good Hope to trade for the spices of the East Indies sickened and died of scurvy.

Under the 'imperialism' heading we can see smallpox and measles spearheading the Spanish conquest of the Aztec and Inca empires and slaughtering so many natives that the Iberians turned to Africa for labor to colonize the Americas. But with African slaves came African diseases such as yellow fever, dengue fever and *falciparum* malaria to enlarge the already swollen pool of pathogens in the Americas and kill still more Indians.

Many diseases are associated with war because, wherever soldiers were drawn together from diverse places in circumstances that were less than hygienic, the tinder was present for epidemic conflagration. Yellow fever was a more fearsome opponent in the West Indies than all of Europe's admirals and generals combined; and it defeated more than a few of them. Typhoid has been a curse of military organizations since battles were fought with clubs and stones; the plague frequently travelled with armies and their followers. And the last two illnesses to be treated in this section – a plague and a pox – are inextricably linked to war: typhus because it has killed far more soldiers and sailors than have killed one another; and syphilis, because it burst upon the world from a battlefield.

Most of these diseases, and the damage they did, flowed from a continuation of human progress. As cities grew larger and their denizens immunologically sturdier, they became especially dangerous to their neighbors. In the fourteenth century Europe was once again fused with the fountain of plague as well as the trade of the east. In the fifteenth century humans perfected the technology that could send men to sea for long periods of time to explore, trade and develop scurvy. By the end of that century the Iberians had taken advantage of progress in map-making, shipbuilding, sail-making and navigation to reach the Americas; and soon after, Old World diseases rained down on the Americans. In the following centuries the ships

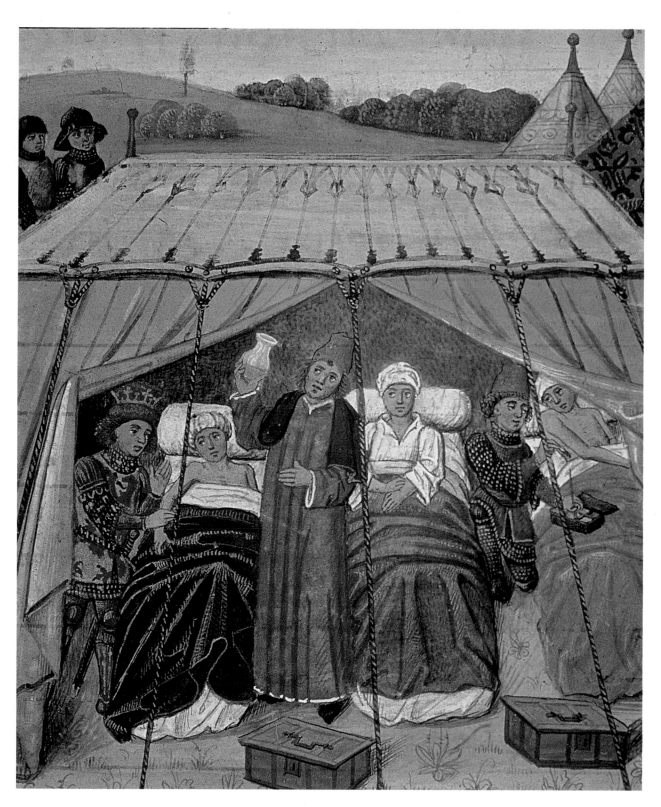

were made faster – sufficiently swift to deliver a cargo of slaves to the New World with minimal loss of life and to transport African pathogens and their vectors intact as well.

Many viewed the extension of European rule over 'heathen' subjects as progress at a time when the 'civilizing' countries were squaring off on battlefields in Europe and all around the globe. It is worthy of note that the observance of the 500th anniversary of the first voyage of Columbus a few years ago did not stimulate joyous celebration among native Americans.

'Care of the Injured: Pulse and urine diagnosis.' (Fifteenth century, from 'Bon Roi Alexandre', Paris.)

The word 'plague' comes from the Latin *plaga*, meaning a strike or a blow that wounds. Before the pandemic of bubonic plague in the 1330s and 1340s, a great plague was believed to reveal God's will, whether His punishment for sin or His plan for the world. Mechanisms to understand the timing, meaning or other particulars of a plague emphasized its spiritual and celestial origins. But the Black Death changed all that. From then onward, at least among European Christians, the focus increasingly turned toward the body, the terrestrial, the victims, the stricken ones. A lawyer in Piacenza, northern Italy, who survived the Black Death provides a good illustration of the subtle shift in emphasis. Gabriele de' Mussis wrote his 'History of the Great Mortality' in the early 1350s, in order to make sense of the catastrophic death toll, a sign of God's displeasure with sinful humanity, and to teach other survivors that order, meaning and redemption were still possible. He provided an account of the plague's origin: the Tartar army was laying siege to Genoese merchants in Kaffa when the plague caught up with it. De' Mussis tells us that the commanders 'ordered corpses to be placed in catapults and lobbed into the city... What seemed like mountains of dead were thrown into the city.' The survivors took to their boats and returned to Europe, bringing the plague with them.

A veteran Muslim traveller named Ibn Battuta simultaneously recorded his near escapes from plague as he journeyed through Persia, Damascus, Cairo and home to west Africa. Venice, Genoa, Cairo and Valencia were all stricken at about the same time. During 1346 and 1347 plague advanced toward Europe simultaneously across the Asian steppes and along Muslim trade routes far to the south.

Crafting his story from travelers' and merchants' tales, the stationary De' Mussis emphasized the role of putrefying bodies in polluting the air and waters of Kaffa. According to both De' Mussis and the Sicilian chronicler Michele da Piazza, the Genoese carried the disease home in their bodies like a portable poison. According to most European witnesses to the Black Death, the first distinctive signs of the new pestilence were the buboes, blotches, boils and pustules seen on the body. Because of these sudden and abnormal swellings on different places of the victims' bodies, we can now confidently identify the epidemic's cause as *Yersinia pestis*. There is no other disease that characteristically produces acute enlargement of the regional lymph nodes, visible in the groin, under the arms, in the neck or behind the ears. For a classic example, consider Giovanni Boccaccio's description of the plague in Florence from the introduction to the *Decameron*, written just after the plague:

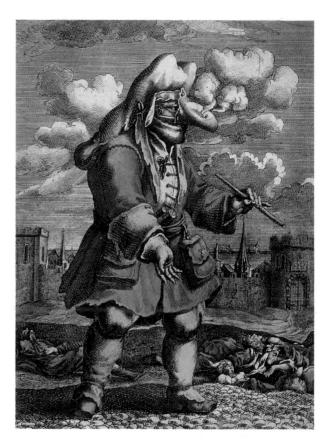

'... its earliest symptom, in men and women alike, was the appearance of certain swellings in the groin or the armpit, some of which were egg-shaped whilst others were roughly the size of the common apple. Sometimes the swellings were large, sometimes not so large, and they were referred to by the populace as *gavòccioli* ... Later on, the symptoms of the disease changed, and many people began to find dark blotches and bruises on their arms, thighs, and other parts of the body, sometimes large and few in number, at other times tiny and closely spaced.'

During the second half of the fourteenth century bubonic plague returned at least four times to most Mediterranean urban centers, and it would recur in Europe every generation for the next three centuries. Beginning with the second epidemic wave (1360–64), chroniclers make direct and specific comparison to the great pestilence of 1348 not because of the high mortality, not because of 'astrological origins' (comets and planetary conjunctions), not because of the problems in managing the crisis, but because the victims had buboes on their bodies. A new plague would be called a pestilence of *anguinaia* (with buboes) and specifically linked to the plague of 1348.

Some pertinent modern biological facts of buboes are in order. *Yersinia pestis* is a bacterium that usually infects rodents and their fleas. In some rodents – for example, the large, gray Norway rat and the Siberian marmot – the animal is ill but able to move and transmit the infection to others. Typically the fleas feeding on the rodents spread the

CHAPTER 9

BUBONIC PLAGUE: THE BLACK DEATH

BY ANN G. CARMICHAEL

disease within rodent colonies, but *Y. pestis* can survive in empty rodent warrens, lying in wait for new victims. *Y. pestis* can also survive in a frozen corpse for years, and in a decaying carcass for a couple of days.

Humans acquire *Y. pestis* infection indirectly when the microorganism reaches nearby rodents that are highly susceptible to the disease. Rats, mice, meadow voles and even rabbits living in proximity to humans are quickly killed by yersinia infection. Fleas then abandon the dying animals in search of friskier hosts. The most likely explanation for the bubonic Black Death of 1348 and subsequent human bubonic plagues is that the black or brown rat (*Rattus rattus*), ubiquitous in Europe, was a ready victim to the spreading plague. The typical flea of that rodent, *Xenopsylla cheopis*, then ensured subsequent human infection for two reasons. First, *X. cheopis* feeds on both human and rodent blood; second, it has a curve or bend in its forestomach or proventriculus, creating a tiny pouch where blood collects and coagulates, a perfect culture plate for *Y. pestis*.

Once bitten by an infected flea, humans have little effective immunity to microbial multiplication. Cells in the area of the bite die quickly, creating a blackening necrotic pustule or blister. Witnesses often refer to this as a plague pustule, 'token', *carbone* or *charbon*. The lymphatic system next drains debris and bacilli to the regional lymph node, a first step in manufacturing a specific antibody. Typically, however, *Y. pestis* grows faster than the human body can contain the infection, and the lymph node swells impressively to the size of an orange or apple, as Boccaccio says. From flea bite to bubo a mere four to six days goes by. When the bubo appears, the bacilli are already reproducing throughout the body, causing high fever, excruciating headache and delirium. Within

ten days, 60 percent of those infected will have died: more than twice the case fatality rates for virulent smallpox and epidemic typhus – and in half the time.

The Black Death killed many – perhaps as many as 20 percent of a Eurasian population estimated at 100 million – and killed with unimaginable speed during the peak of the epidemic. Soaring death rates prevented any semblance of normal burial practice. Eyewitness accounts described mounds of rotting cadavers and the inability of collecting, much less burying the bodies. Boccaccio and others described these lugubrious scenes in order to impress on posterity the enormity of this mortality, and to reflect upon the breakdown of social customs and mores during the epidemic. Later plague chroniclers did not specifically compare their own burial crises with those of the Black Death, but they clearly anticipated similar problems in managing dead bodies, even as mere rumors of plague arrive. Local losses of 40 to 50 percent were not uncommon.

When the plague hit, mortality soared. Because some of those bitten by infected fleas develop a secondary plague pneumonia, or lung infection, the organism can be coughed directly on to anyone close by. In this airborne form, *Y. pestis*

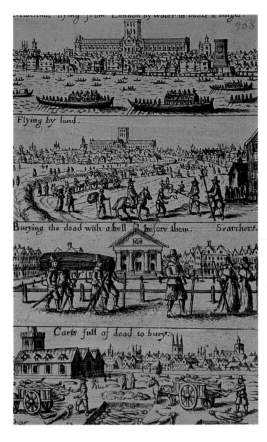

Plague of London. 1665 woodcut. Magdalene College, Cambridge.

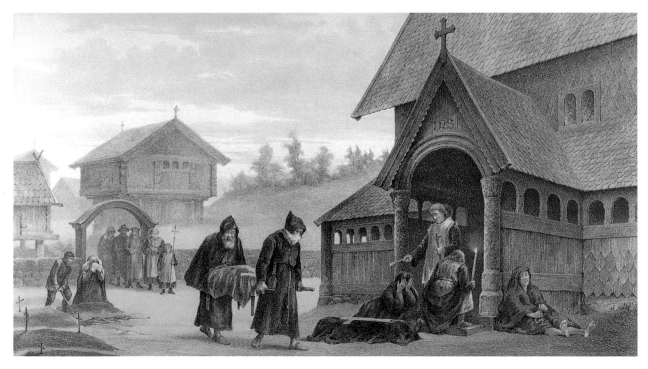

The Black Death of 1349 killed off two in three of Norway's population.

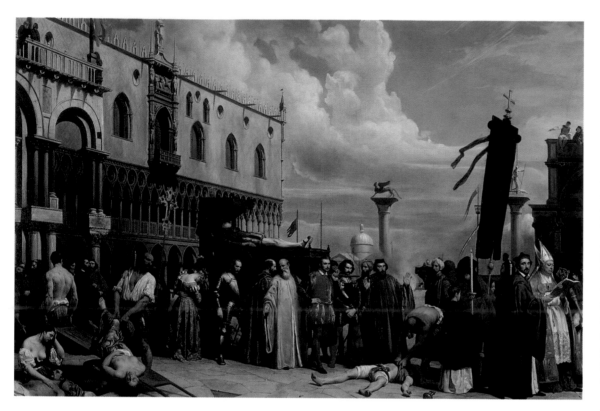

Funerary honours given to Titian, who died in Venice in the Plague of 1576. (Painted by Alexandre-Jean-Baptiste Hesse (1806–79), in 1832.)

cheese between layers of lasagna'. The Black Death was unprecedented both in the numbers of bodies to bury and in the appearance of the corpses at death. Attention to the physical management of human bodies before and after death became the focus of plague controls for the centuries to come.

During the great plague Jews were deemed capable of deliberately spreading the plague from place to place, while remaining unaffected themselves. Though the Greek historian Thucydides had accused the Spartans of deliberate biological warfare by poisoning the wells of Athens in 430 BC, the Black Death saw the first modern claims of *pestis manufacta* (human-caused plague) and the subsequent tortures, confessions and pogroms. So the Black Death sets the measure for all other pestilences – it is the gold standard of killer epidemics.

is nearly always fatal, producing primary pneumonic plague. For example, in a city the size of Florence (roughly 100,000 before the Black Death), one or two hundred deaths occurred every day through the late spring; then suddenly 400 to 1,000 died every day.

The biology and epidemiology of human plague help to explain how so many could die and why the die-off suddenly sky-rocketed, but it is the medieval chroniclers who convey the horror of the visible, physical presence of massive numbers of unburied bodies. A Florentine born in 1349, Marchione di Coppo Stefani, wrote that bodies were thrown into newly dug trenches in hastily consecrated ground, and dirt sprinkled between the layers of limbs and torsos 'like

Several library shelves could be filled with the studies of the causes, effects and consequences of this one great plague. But some attention to the periodic recurrences of plague in Europe is necessary. From 1347 until 1722, plague returned regularly to western Europe, and without the help of Arabian trebuchets. The last large epidemic was that of Marseille, in 1720, by which time most regions of Europe had been plague-free for over half a century. Led by Italian city states, during the intervening period Europeans developed a range of new, plague-related practices that form the foundations of modern epidemic surveillance and control. Earliest of these was the maritime quarantine devised in 1377 in the Venetian colony of Ragusa (now Dubrovnik, in Croatia). The first quarantine was a *trentino*, of thirty days, but like later forty-

In the Plague of 1630, townspeople try to escape to the country. A Looking Glass for Town and Country – *contemporary broadside.*

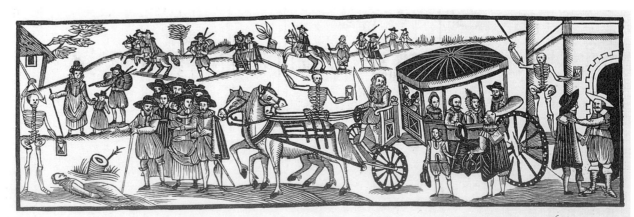

FLIGHT OF THE TOWNSPEOPLE INTO THE COUNTRY TO ESCAPE FROM THE PLAGUE, A.D. 1630
" A Looking-glass for Town and Country ;" broadside in the collection of the Society of Antiquaries.

day quarantines, its purpose was to prevent importation of disease, rather than to isolate individuals already ill.

Quarantine for inland areas was far more difficult to manage. Italian cities endangered by plague developed a form of health passport crafted for moneyed, literate travelers at their points of origin, to certify their plague-free status. This maneuver, designed initially to lessen the burdens of temporary confinement, required an efficient bureaucracy. Boards of health quickly assumed other plague tasks, namely isolation of the ill, separate quarantine/isolation of those who had had contact with the sick, management of the medical, philanthropic and burial services needed during the epidemic and, above all, record-keeping. Recurrent plagues prompted records of deaths and causes of death, networks of spies to provide an intelligence surveillance system, the design and management of confinement hospitals, letter writing and routine diplomacy on behalf of privileged travelers, and inventories of confiscated or destroyed properties. Not only was plague terribly expensive in human lives, it was almost as costly as warfare for societies that had limited, non-renewable bases of wealth. But it was also an undeniable stimulus to the growth of the modern bureaucratic state.

In retrospect it seems most likely that *Y. pestis* was continually imported to Europe, principally via Mediterranean trade. However, subsequent large epidemics did not spread over Europe, as did the Black Death, like ripples from a large stone dropped into a pond. The existence of regional foci, where yersinia was established among rodent colonies, would best explain the continual flare-ups in areas far removed from maritime trade. For example, several large epidemics approached the large inland city of Milan simultaneously through the alpine passes to the north and east, along the Po river through northern Italy, or along traditional north–south pilgrimage routes linking France, the low countries, and England with Rome. Thus the choke-hold of plague on Europe could not be loosened solely through maritime quarantine.

Nonetheless plague did disappear from Europe after the seventeenth century; there were only two large epidemics after 1670. Though the last episodes of plague in Europe were nearly as virulent as the Black Death, the microbe did not succeed in maintaining enzootic plague in the animal population. In fact, Europe is

the only continent that nowadays has no naturally occurring *Y. pestis* in rodents.

There is considerable historical speculation about the reasons for the plague's disappearance. Among these the development of rodent immunity or the introduction of less susceptible rodents to Europe seem the least likely, for rodents with higher resistance to plague create stable niches for enzootic yersinia. The most attractive hypotheses are that human ingenuity or effort stanched the transmission of infection through trade between the Middle East and Europe. Maritime quarantines, for example, could have decreased the number of plague rats and fleas reaching western Europe. The expansion of north Atlantic, and then global, oceanic trade in the seventeenth century circumvented the traditional trade routes to the east, and may thus have taken the wind out of the plague's sails. Finally, the appearance of an odorless, tasteless arsenical rat bane in the second half of the seventeenth century may have been effective in reducing susceptible rodent populations outside the Mediterranean.

It is also possible, however, that human agency had little to do with the major cause of the plague's disappearance. The reign of Louis XIV, the 'Sun King', corresponded with a

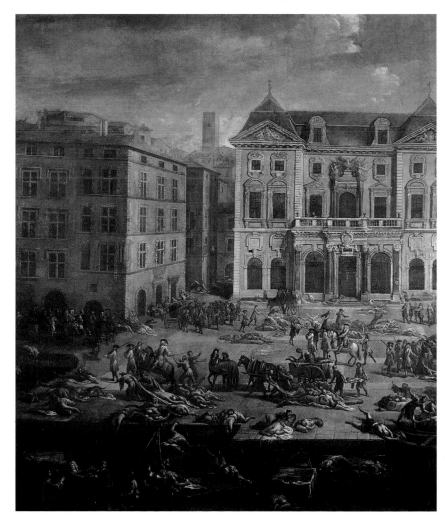

View of the Town Hall, Marseilles, during the Plague of 1721. (Michel Serre, 1658–1753). Musée des Beaux-Arts, Marseilles.

The Great Fire of London which, by killing infected rats, cleansed the city of bubonic plague.

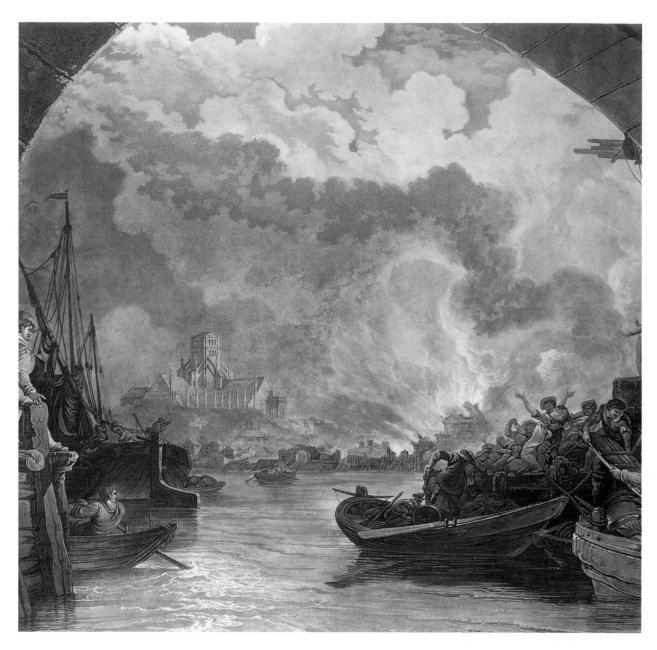

period of low sunspot activity, globally cooler temperatures and the advance of glaciers. It could be that these momentous ecological events led to changes in the migratory patterns of Eurasian rodents, and in turn restricted the dissemination of plague. Recurrent plague also effected considerable demographic and economic damage to Muslim societies, and it is possible that the thinning of human populations in the plague regions of central Asia simultaneously decreased the number of times that the plague inoculum reached the West and the extent of the damage.

Europeans nevertheless continued to expect the plague's return, stepping up quarantine and isolation efforts, and improving their diagnosis of cases of bubonic plague. In 1720, for example, plague reached Marseille, presumably through failures in the long-practiced quarantine system. A

Levantine boat on which cases of human plague appeared in the spring of 1720 was refused disembarkation at Livorno and Marseille, but rerouted the cargo, passengers and crew through Tripoli, to obtain an equivocal bill of health. When it returned to Toulon in July, officials there imposed a perfunctory quarantine, but many aboard were able to bribe their way to liberty. Soon afterwards plague flared in Toulon, the poorer neighborhoods of Marseille, and in smaller towns to the north and east, along the frequently travelled roads.

We cannot be as sure as the contemporary accounts would have it that the cargo and crew of one ship carrying cotton were responsible for the great plague that followed. Over 50,000 died, of a Marseille population of around 100,000. By September and October the plague so overwhelmed local resources that bodies piled up everywhere. Some of the most

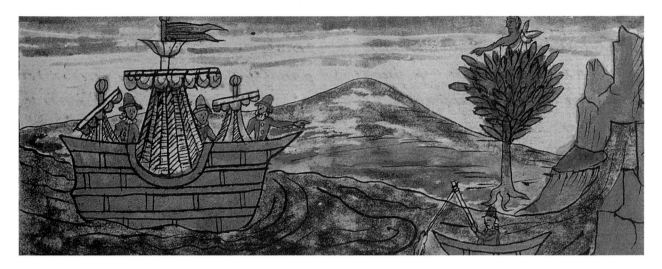

An Indian spy observes the arrival of Spanish sailors on the Mexican coast, from a 1518 manuscript by Diego Duran, Historia de las Indias.

horrific of plague stories lingered long in popular memory: the chevalier Roze imposed draconian order, chasing away prowling dogs with gun blasts, drafting all the available soldiers and convicts to clear passageways, though some of the cadavers had been dead for more than ten days. Roze himself had to steel his troops by dismounting and hoisting some of the most putrefied bodies over his shoulders.

News of the unfolding catastrophe in Marseille quickly spread through Europe, and most notably occasioned Daniel Defoe's fictitious account of the 1665 London plague, *Journal of the Plague Year*. All maritime commerce with Marseille ceased and the provincial government in Provence imposed a strict quarantine in the foothills surrounding the port areas, dispatching physicians and surgeons to replace those who had fled.

The grand medical school of Montpellier sent a team of physicians who commanded separate quarters and quickly became rivals of the few local medical worthies who stayed to fight the plague. The Montpellier clinicians performed autopsies, aspirating liquid from the buboes of victims and injecting the substance experimentally into animals, conducting studies eerily remote from the scenes of disaster in the streets. Of the forty volunteers and one hundred convicts that Roze commanded, five, including Roze himself, survived. Twenty-five of thirty available local surgeons died; most of the local collegiate physicians and four of the seventeen surgeons that the provincial health office had sent fell ill or died from plague. As in all the great plagues of Europe, most of the deaths fell within a two-month period – here mid-August through mid-October.

The events in Marseille were enough to redouble governmental and mercantile reliance on quarantine throughout the eighteenth century, but with increasing focus on constricting or eliminating the Middle Eastern cloth trade. Conveniently the threat of plague facilitated western European global colonization and economic

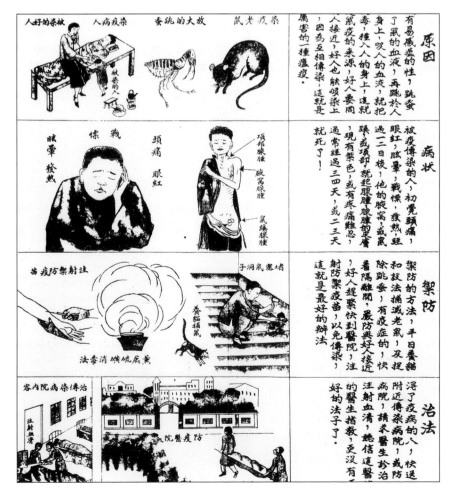

This Chinese poster, made in September 1930 after the great Manchurian pneumonic plague, educates viewers and readers about the causes, manifestations, preventions, and treatments of bubonic plague.

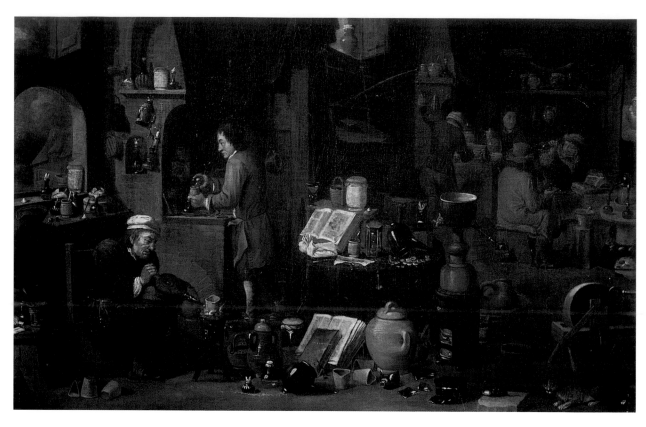

development. Non-Europeans were seen to be such a threat that the Austrian-Hungarian Empire invested in a 1,500-mile *cordon sanitaire* stretching overland from the Balkans to north of the Danube, with guard houses so closely spaced that guards could stay in visual contact with one another.

Naturally, the guards were not looking for rats or fleas, so the investment did little to stop the spread of plague. Trade routes redirected through central Russia, from the Crimea and the Caspian Sea up the Volga to Moscow and St Petersburg, brought plague to Moscow in 1770–71 an epidemic as devastating as that of Marseille a half-century earlier. Plague did not extend over the same territory during the early nineteenth century, however, even with the building of railroads and the expansion of overland trade that brought Asiatic cholera to Moscow in the late 1820s.

A recent painstaking study of the gradual spread of plague through Yunnan, China, down the West and Red River valleys to the sea, provides an insight into the slow passage of plague through rugged rural terrain and along minor, even contraband, trade routes. Plague in China did not require the European *Rattus rattus* species; the yellow-chested rat, *Rattus flavipectus*, an indigenous rodent in seventeen of twenty-six south Chinese provinces, was equally susceptible to plague. Though Chinese sources do not provide good records of the sporadic epidemics in the mountainous hinterlands, it has been shown that plague moved from the mining towns of western Yunnan to local prefecture centers of the Ching dynasty. But the Opium Wars with Britain in the1840s, then the Taiping and Muslim rebellions in the interior, in the

1850s and 1860s respectively, severely disrupted the passage of tea, opium and other highly profitable items along the West River. The central Ching government, faced with mounting military costs and epidemic opium usage, increased tariffs along the West river, thereby making tedious overland trade more competitive; by the late 1880s plague epidemics marched toward new trading ports, especially Behai, and along the Mekong and Red Rivers through Southeast Asia.

By 1894 plague had reached Hong Kong and Canton, and by 1896, Bombay. As in 1348, plague moved along many trade fronts simultaneously, abetted in its spread by changing volume of trade, warfare, and characteristic urban disinterest in the depopulation of rural hinterlands. Plague became visible only when it hit urban areas or compromised profits. Interestingly, Chinese descriptions of the plague, unlike those of westerners, noted the preceding mortality of rats. For example, a poem by Shi Doanan in the late 1790s speaks of 'strange rats' coming out of the ground during the daytime, spitting up blood and falling down dead. Humans were said to die in great numbers from 'breathing the odor of dead rats' or from seeing them: 'In each family that got sick, the rats first jumped out without any reason, faltered and fell dead in front of people. Those who saw them became sick in a very short while.' Chinese accounts may have drawn westerners' attention to the rats, which are not linked to plague in Europe in early modern times.

When plague reached the great Asian port cities of the late nineteenth century, the entire western world was on alert. Alexandre Yersin, a former student and laboratory assistant at the Pasteur Institute in Paris, was in French Indochina when plague reached Hong Kong. With a translator and an assistant he raced there, arriving three days after a Japanese delegation led by Shibasaburo Kitasato. Trained originally in Robert Koch's Berlin laboratories, Kitasato had already secured access to all plague patients and cadavers. Yersin constructed a straw hut on the grounds of the Alice Memorial Hospital and from there bribed gravediggers to let corpses linger in a shed long enough for him to obtain samples from the buboes and organs of the victims. Both men published their reports speedily in European journals, but in retrospect it is clear that Yersin unambiguously described the organism that now bears his name. Moreover Yersin noted the unusual mortality of rats, and the ease with which rats and mice could be infected with the organism he had cultured from buboes. Thus by late 1894 the microbial cause of plague was identified and the triumph published globally through international medical journals.

The Tenth International Sanitary Conference, which met in Venice in 1897, was devoted to plague. Britain, Prussia, Austria-Hungary, Italy, Russia and France all dispatched plague investigators to the scenes of south Asian plagues. Within the year the British Indian Plague Commission proved the rat's role in the transmission of plague, but assumed that rat-to-rat transmission occurred through rats eating their fallen comrades. They thus speculated that poor sanitation was largely to blame.

Unfortunately western response to the widening, accelerating plague in India in the late 1890s was to enforce draconian isolation of the victims and their contacts, to burn clothing and cadavers, to fumigate houses and to raze slum accommodations, despite the mounting bacteriological evidence that questioned such a strategy.

Meanwhile plague had also spread throughout the Pacific rim, notably to Sydney and to San Francisco in 1900. Sydney's public health and medical officers brought plague under control by 1902 by destroying the rodent population around the wharves. The San Francisco authorities, on the other hand, forced the quarantine of over 20,000 Asian immigrants in Chinatown, imposing trade and travel restrictions on selective, racial criteria. The Chinese immigrants also became 'volunteer' recipients of Waldemar Haffkine's anti-plague vaccine.

The introduction of yersinia to rodent colonies in the continents of Australia, North America, South America and southern Africa dates from this late nineteenth-century pandemic, effectively establishing foci of enzootic and epizootic plague everywhere on the globe except Europe. Plague epidemics in the twentieth century have nevertheless replicated past patterns, being associated most with imperialism and warfare.

BIBLIOGRAPHY

Arnold, David. 1993. *Colonizing the Body: State Medicine and Epidemic Disease in Nineteenth-Century India.* Berkeley, California and London.
Benedict, Carol. 1996. *Bubonic Plague in Nineteenth-Century China.* Stanford.
Biraben, Jean Noël. 1975. *Les Hommes et la peste en France et dans les Pays Européens et Méditerranéens* (2 vols). Paris.
Hirst, Lucian Fabian. 1953. *The Conquest of Plague: a Study of the Evolution of Epidemiology.* Oxford.
Horrox, Rosemary (ed. and trans.) 1994. *The Black Death.* Manchester and New York.
Mollaret, H. H. and J. Brossolet. 1985. *Alexandre Yersin, le vainqueur de la peste.* Paris.
Slack, Paul. 1985. *The Plague in Tudor and Stuart England.* London.

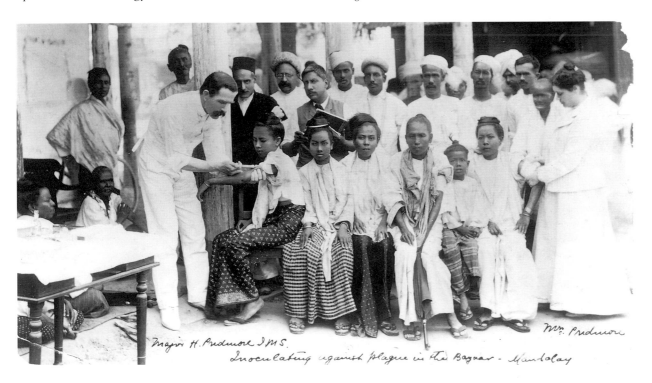

Major H. Predmore IMS.
Inoculating against plague in the Bazaar - Mandalay

Mr. Predmore

Major H. Predmore, inoculating against plague in the bazaar, Mandalay, Burma

CHAPTER 10

SCURVY: CITRUS AND SAILORS

By Stephen V. Beck

Scurvy, the 'scourge of sailors', for long a medical mystery, is now known to be a nutritional deficiency disease. Although it has killed many people throughout history, scurvy poses little danger today. As long as it is properly and speedily diagnosed, it is completely curable.

Early French explorers called scurvy '*mal de terre*', and slave traders later called it *mal de Luanda*. But the term 'scurvy' itself goes back only to early modern times, its roots lying in words like the Danish *scorbuck*, the Dutch *schverbaujck* and the Saxon *schorbock*, which were given a Latinized form, *scorbutus*, in 1541.

Scurvy is caused by a deficiency of vitamin C (ascorbic acid) in the diet. Unlike most mammals, humans do not synthesize vitamin C in their bodies, and thus must obtain it from a diet that includes fresh fruits and vegetables, the richest sources of vitamin C. Although dangerous and deadly if not treated, scurvy advances relatively slowly, and can be reversed by consumption of vitamin C at virtually any point in the progress of the disease. In our century the symptoms have been well documented by a number of experiments involving volunteers who induced the condition in themselves through deliberate restriction to a scorbutic, or scurvy-causing, diet.

After about three months with no vitamin C, the sufferer begins to feel tired and listless. Within another two months, the skin is affected, first becoming rough and dry; by around the end of the sixth month, hemorrhages in the legs appear and wounds will not heal. At seven and a half months the victim's gums soften, swell and turn purple – historical sources add that teeth became loose as well, and that old wounds opened up again. The condition appears to become life-threatening in the period between seven and nine and a half months; some voluntary sufferers have developed cardiac and pulmonary difficulties during this span.

Scurvy may strike in any situation that subjects people to a scorbutic diet, which has frequently occurred when food supplies must come from afar. But historically the disease has been most closely associated with sailors spending lengthy periods at sea; estimates suggest that, between 1600 and 1800, scurvy killed more than one million sailors – more, probably, than all the deaths from shipwrecks, naval warfare and other diseases combined. It has also attacked soldiers and others during large-scale or prolonged wars and, like most of the nutritional deficiency diseases, has been a particular scourge of the inmates of institutions – hospital patients, prison convicts, confined lunatics and the like. Scurvy can be especially dangerous in colder areas of the world where dietary sources of vitamin C are less plentiful and varied; thus, another peculiarly susceptible group has been explorers of the arctic regions.

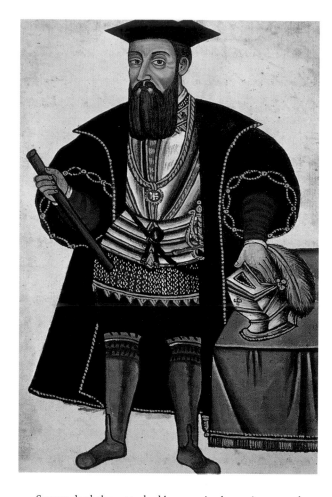

Vasco da Gama, Portuguese navigator, and the first westerner to sail round the Cape of Good Hope to Asia. Illustration by Pedro Barretti de Resende, 1646.

Scurvy doubtless attacked humans in the ancient past, but it is not certain whether they viewed it as a disease entity in its own right, and thus it is difficult to pick out clear references to scurvy in ancient texts. The Egyptian Ebers papyrus, from around 1500 BC, contains what may be a description of scurvy. Likewise, Hippocratic medical writings from the fifth century BC in ancient Greece refer to certain symptoms that could indicate the disease. Roman soldiers in areas such as northern Europe may have suffered from scurvy once they were removed from the varied diet of the Mediterranean region.

A number of thirteenth-century sources suggest that the Crusaders may have been affected by scurvy while fighting in the Near East. Another document from the same period advises those traveling on board ship to include fruits and vegetables in their baggage. Later medieval texts do not mention scurvy specifically, although there are many references to loosened teeth that may signify the presence of the disease.

In the earliest stages of the 'Age of Exploration', the prolonged ocean voyages of the late fifteenth and early sixteenth centuries – made feasible by new navigation techniques and shipbuilding technology – first established scurvy in the European mind as a distinct and recognizable disease. First the Portuguese and then the Spaniards – later followed by men from other nations – sailed out into the

Atlantic, often for months at a time, and, inevitably, scurvy became a part of shipboard life – and death.

A more scorbutic diet than that consumed by these early sailors can scarcely be imagined. They subsisted on salted, dried or smoked meats and fish, old cheese, hardtack (a dense, dry biscuit), dried legumes, and water or beer. Fresh fruits or vegetables could sometimes be obtained when a ship made landfall, but this was usually infrequent, and anyway such fare did not keep more than a few days on board ship.

During the fifteenth century, Portuguese mariners worked their way down the west coast of Africa, establishing ports for supplies and trade and learning to negotiate the strange winds and currents of the South Atlantic. This effort culminated in 1487, when Bartolomeu Dias rounded the Cape of Good Hope at the southern end of Africa and sailed into the Indian Ocean. Eleven years later the Portuguese captain Vasco da Gama, rounding southern Africa on the way to India, recorded what may be the first clear description of scurvy. His fleet's company was badly afflicted by the disease, and perhaps as many as half died of it.

Ferdinand Magellan's crew suffered from scurvy during their 1519 to 1522 voyage that completed the first circumnavigation of the earth. At Tierra del Fuego, the men fought the disease by eating wild celery, and they also began eating rats, animals now known to produce their own vitamin C. In 1523 a French expedition along the North American coast fell victim to scurvy, as did the party under the command of Jacques Cartier, who, during his discovery and exploration of the St Lawrence River between 1534 and 1536, lost a number of his crew to the disease and recorded a much-quoted description of the symptoms. Cartier and his companions learned from the Indians they encountered of a local remedy for the

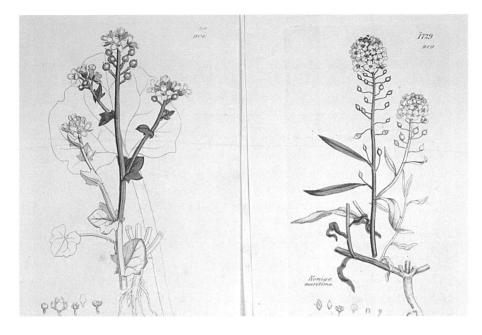

condition, 'spruce beer'. It was brewed from the bark and leaves of evergreens and, though some of the men were reluctant to drink it, apparently proved an efficacious cure. Some forty years later, during Francis Drake's circumnavigation of the globe between 1577 and 1580, a beverage concocted from tree leaves and bark was again used to treat scurvy.

'Humoral' theories of medicine had prevailed for some hundreds of years by the mid-sixteenth century, and contemporary physicians designated scurvy as a disease caused by an excess of the 'melancholic' humor, black bile, which in turn had resulted from a failure of the spleen to

A 1799 depiction of 'scurvy grass,' or spoonwort (Cochlearia officinalis). For centuries, it was considered the most effective specific against scurvy, but the plant actually contains relatively little vitamin C.

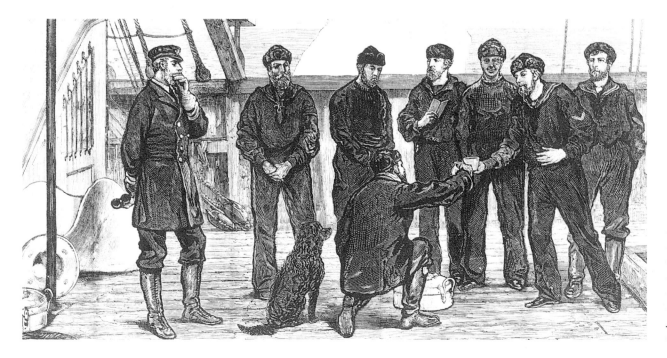

Because their diet usually lacked variey, Arctic explorers were at risk of scurvy. Here, crewmen of the Alert, in 1875, receive their daily ration of lime juice to ward off the disease.

regulate properly the level of black bile in the body. The malfunction of the spleen, however, was presumed by many to arise from a dietary cause.

The plant, *Cochlearia officinalis*, also called 'scurvy grass' or spoonwort, was a favored treatment for scurvy, from about the 1500s to the 1700s, but we now know that it actually has a relatively low content of vitamin C. In addition to 'scurvy grass', watercress and 'brooklime' were much favored by Europeans of the sixteenth, seventeenth and eighteenth centuries. All three were grown specifically as remedies for scurvy, but it is not known how or when these plants developed their antiscorbutic reputation.

Throughout the sixteenth century, developing navigational and shipbuilding technology on the one hand, and intense competition for colonies and trade on the other, meant that the merchant fleets, exploration vessels and navies of the European nations made more – and longer – voyages, and the grip of scurvy upon the ships' crews did not slacken. Then, in 1601, the British East India Company sent a trading fleet to Sumatra. It was at sea for over seven months before even reaching southern Africa, and the crew of every ship but one was laid low by scurvy. The one exception was the vessel carrying Sir James Lancaster, who had provisioned his sailors with oranges and lemons. This was reportedly one of the first times that these fruits were employed preemptively against the disease.

By the end of the sixteenth century, many people were aware that fresh foods in general, and citrus fruits in particular, seemed to work almost miraculous cures on sailors

Frobisher's men in a skirmish with Eskimos at Bloody Point. Despite the lack of fruit and vegetables in their diet, Eskimos did not get scurvy because of the large amounts of raw or semi-cooked meat that they ate.

suffering from scurvy. But limes or lemons were not readily available to the nations of northern Europe (which were beginning to dominate the competition for sea power) nor were the fruits easily transported on long voyages because they were perishable – a problem which would eventually lead to the development of concentrated fruit juice. But even if the fruits had been preservable, naval vessels in particular had a problem: their companies were becoming simply too large to be adequately provisioned with them. In addition – perhaps the most difficult obstacle to overcome – medical theories of scurvy did not necessarily accept the practical observations that citrus fruits cured or prevented it.

Many people continued to seek other cures for scurvy, either because they disbelieved the efficacy of citrus fruits or because they hoped to substitute for them something less perishable and less expensive. Nevertheless, during the seventeenth century, the Dutch planted citrus orchards on islands along the ocean route around Africa. They also experimented with gardening on board ship, but the gardens were frequently overwhelmed by high seas. The Hudson's Bay Company regularly sent lime juice to North America, where scurvy worked to obstruct the colonization of parts of Canada.

As the European navies grew in power and prestige, their sailors probably fared worse with scurvy than those serving in merchant ships. In the navies, both the length of time spent at sea and the regular making of ports-of-call were dictated by the ships' military role, and certainly were scheduled less systematically than in trading fleets. By the mid-eighteenth century such factors had become so important that they contributed to what has been called one of the worst medical disasters at sea in history.

Between 1740 and 1744 British Commodore George Anson circumnavigated the globe on a mission against Spanish shipping in the Pacific. The voyage was described as a success, but Anson lost 1,855 men out of his original complement of 2,000; numerous causes of death were listed, but most of the sailors had died of scurvy. (A Spanish fleet that pursued Anson's was reported to have lost 2,900 of its 3,000 men.) Anson would later become First Lord of the Admiralty and appoint James Lind, the father of the modern approach to scurvy, as chief physician of the Haslar naval hospital.

Around the same time as Anson's circumnavigation, British naval surgeon Edward Ives tried using cider (because of the scarcity of citrus fruits) to prevent scurvy and found that it kept his crewmen healthy, although they did develop scurvy after the cider ran out. Wishing to test Ives's success with cider, James Lind set up a shipboard experiment in 1747 with six groups of scorbutic sailors. He gave citrus fruits to

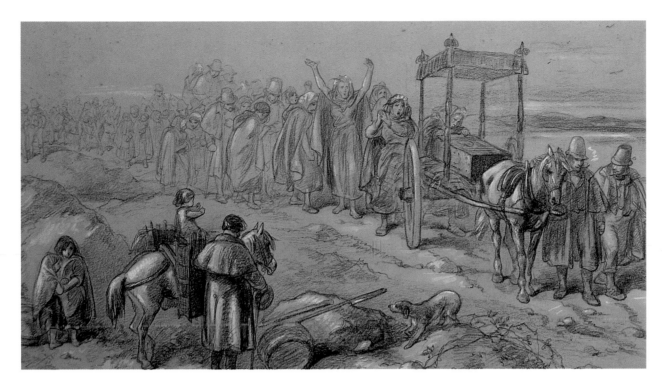

Irish funeral. Chalk and pencil drawing by John Doyle (1797–1868). The potato famine of the 1840s led to much scurvy, as well as starvation.

one group, cider to another, and various other substances to the remainder. Only those who received citrus fruits recovered their full health.

Some have claimed that Lind's experiment constituted the first controlled clinical trial in the history of medicine. Whether or not this was the case, his shipboard tests, which he described in his 1753 book, *A Treatise on the Scurvy*, proved that citrus juices could cure the disease. Lind himself argued that a number of measures and treatments – the use of citrus fruits among them – would prevent or cure it. Actually, he thought that beer was the best anti-scorbutic, but it could not be preserved well and was inconvenient to carry. For purposes of storage and transportation, he recommended juicing citrus fruits and condensing the juice into citrus 'rob', a syrupy substance. In corked bottles it would keep for some years, even on board ship, and could be reconstituted much as we add water to frozen orange juice concentrate today.

At the time, however, other theories as well as Lind's were in vogue. Although some in the medical profession (and others outside it) agreed that citrus fruits were successful in treating scurvy, many believed that other remedies would work just as well. Moreover, the high cost of citrus fruits continued to make cheaper substitutes preferable. Many agreed with Lind's belief that beer or other malt beverages were efficacious anti-scorbutics, and, in 1776,

Captain James Cook recommended malt instead of citrus juice; the use of malt – already popular – was continued.

But Sir Gilbert Blane, another naval physician, appointed to the Board of Sick and Wounded Sailors in 1795, renewed the argument for the use of lime or lemon juice. By the end of the eighteenth century, the Royal Navy finally made it a regular part of sailors' rations, each man receiving three-quarters of an ounce daily. As a result, the threat of scurvy was largely removed from British sailors, although the crewmen of foreign navies and others on land were not so fortunate.

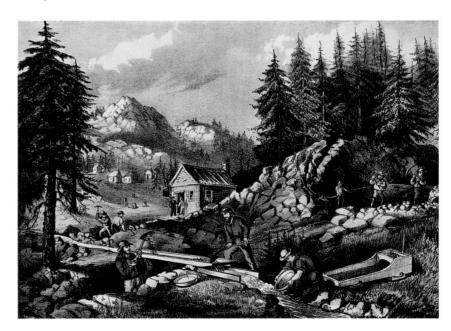

Goldmining in California, 1871, N. Currier and J. M. Ives. Scurvy struck those in remote goldfields in the California Gold Rush of 1848.

Chinese doctor taking the pulse of a sick man. From a collection on Chinese medicine. Batavia, Seventeenth century.

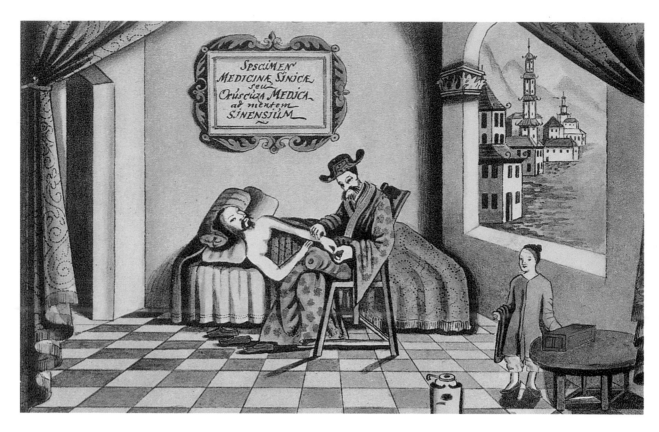

During the Napoleonic Wars, Napoleon's navy suffered greatly from scurvy, and it is likely that his army, especially on its retreat from Russia, was also afflicted with it in addition to typhus. In the early nineteenth century – after the Royal Navy had successfully adopted citrus juices as a preventive measure – scurvy outbreaks continued in British institutions such as prisons or workhouses. These, however, were not widespread and were more or less easily controlled.

It was also during this period that it was first noted that European and American members of arctic expeditions were frequently stricken by scurvy, although natives of the arctic region were not. It has since been discovered that Eskimos have always been generally scurvy-free, despite a lack of fruits and vegetables. This is because of the large amounts of fresh meat – much of it eaten raw or semi-cooked – in the Eskimo diet. Fresh meat is a good source of vitamin C, but heat can very quickly destroy it.

In the meantime, the New World potato, brought to Europe in the sixteenth century, had become the primary dietary source of vitamin C for many people. In Ireland and Scotland it was also the staple food, so that the Irish potato famine of the 1840s led to much scurvy as well as starvation. Unfortunately, the grains sent by the British government to relieve the situation contained no vitamin C, and the disease consequently reached epidemic proportions in both countries.

In 1846 American sailors blockading Mexico during its war with the United States suffered from scurvy, and during the California Gold Rush of 1848 the disease struck among those in remote goldfields surviving on a poor diet. British and French soldiers in the Crimean War of 1854 to 1856, and possibly Turkish troops as well, were afflicted when their supply lines were cut. The disease was rampant during the American Civil War, especially in prisoner-of-war camps – vitamin C deficiency accounting in one case for a 9 percent monthly death rate. Finally, scurvy broke out during the siege of Paris in the Franco-Prussian War of 1870–71.

In addition, beginning at about this time and lasting until World War I, an enduring, widespread epidemic of 'infantile scurvy' (then believed to be a disease different from scurvy) occurred in the United States and Europe – that is, in the industrialized parts of the world. This, as we now know, was the result of mothers (especially among the upper economic classes) eschewing breast-feeding and instead employing the newly invented condensed or evaporated milks or infant formulas, which contained no vitamin C.

Up to this time there had been general agreement that scurvy had a dietary cause, although the prevailing medical theories of previous centuries had varied widely in their analyses of just how this functioned. But in the latter part of the nineteenth century, the development and general acceptance of the germ theory of disease caused a setback in medical thinking about scurvy. Researchers were deflected from seeking a dietary origin and instead searched for a microorganism – or a toxin produced by a microorganism – that caused the disease. Early research into the causes of another nutritional deficiency disease, beriberi, had incorporated a similarly false assumption. But unlike the case of beriberi, in which researchers soon discarded the germ theory and returned to ideas of a dietary cause, scurvy research was badly sidetracked for some thirty years into seeking a bacterial origin for the disease.

Fortunately, around the turn of the twentieth century, the predictions of British physician George Budd began to be fulfilled. In the 1840s Budd had written that scurvy, like some other illnesses, was the result of a diet deficient in a single element, which was present in fruits and vegetables, and that this element would soon be identified by methods of organic chemistry. He could not have stated it better.

In the last years of the nineteenth century and the first years of the twentieth, Norwegian bacteriologist Axel Holst, studying 'ship beriberi' in Norway, wanted to replicate beriberi experiments with chickens that had originally been carried out in Java. By chance, however, he chose to use guinea pigs rather than chickens, both because they were convenient and because they were mammals, and thus more human-like. In 1907 Holst reported that, while the guinea pigs were being test-fed an all-grain diet, they began to show symptoms of scurvy.

In choosing guinea pigs, Holst had unwittingly selected test animals that, like humans, are unable to produce their own vitamin C. Once this was realized, guinea pigs were used to test any potential anti-scorbutic treatment, and they continued in this role up to the time that vitamin C itself was chemically formulated. (There is underway today a search for a mutant guinea pig resistant to scurvy, which could aid research into the possibility of human resistance to the disease.) But Holst's own experiments with the animals strongly indicated the connection between scurvy and diet, and his findings received powerful support in 1912, when Polish-born biochemist Casimir Funk put forward his famous theory of four nutritional deficiency diseases: beriberi, pellagra, rickets and scurvy. Funk posited that in each case a crucial element was absent from the diet; he designated these crucial elements 'vitamines'.

But some bacteriologists continued to resist the notion of dietary deficiencies and 'vitamines' (later shortened to 'vitamins'), especially in the case of scurvy; in one experiment, bacteria taken from scorbutic animals had apparently induced symptoms of scurvy in test animals. Even Elmer V. McCollum, the eventual discoverer of some of the vitamins, held for some time to the theory that the disease was caused by toxins produced in the host body by microorganisms. Adherence to the deficiency theory gained momentum, however, especially during the 1920s, as many advances took place in the search for the vitamins. By 1932 vitamin C had been isolated and chemically identified through the efforts of Hungarian Albert Szent-Györgyi and American Glen King.

Scurvy has been conquered but not eradicated. Nowadays, in developed countries, scurvy can sometimes be seen in single, middle-aged men, who are somewhat at risk of consuming an unbalanced diet if living alone. In developing countries, reports of scurvy are infrequent, but it is difficult to determine whether this is the result of a generally more antiscorbutic diet or merely indicates inadequate medical reporting. Recent Third World victims of the disease have included Ethiopian refugees in Sudan and Somalia, who apparently received vitamin C-deficient relief food in refugee camps. Their suffering is a reminder that humans do not live by bread (or cereals) alone, and that the scourge of scurvy has yet to be eliminated.

BIBLIOGRAPHY

Carpenter, Kenneth J. 1986. *The History of Scurvy and Vitamin C.* Cambridge.

Cuppage, Francis E. 1994. *James Cook and the Conquest of Scurvy.* Westport, Connecticut.

French, Roger K. 1993. 'Scurvy', in Kenneth K. Kiple (ed.), *The Cambridge World History of Human Disease.* Cambridge, England and New York.

Hirsch, August. 1883–6. *Handbook of Geographical and Historical Pathology* (trans. Charles Creighton), 3 vols. London.

A painting depicting the shooting of a prisoner at the Andersonville prisoner-of-war camp during the American Civil War. The prisoners' poor diets made scurvy rife in such prisons, and many died of it.

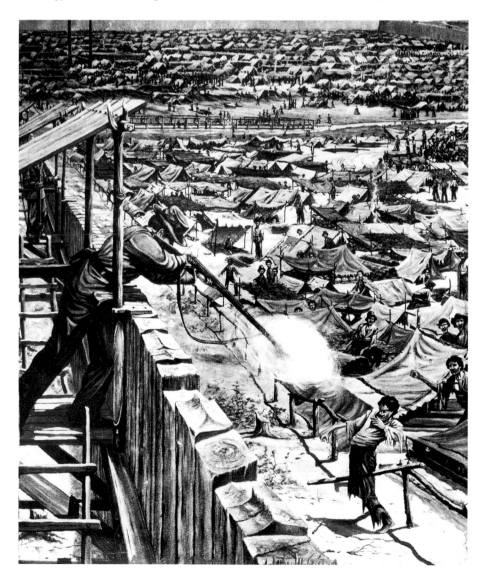

CHAPTER 11

SMALLPOX: 'THERE NEVER WAS A CURE'

By Alfred Crosby

Smallpox was called *small*pox to differentiate it from the great pox or syphilis, but whatever the diameter of its pustules as compared to those of the venereal infection, the former disease had by far the greater influence on human affairs. There were two kinds of the disease in the last century, *variola major* and *variola minor*, the former with a death rate of perhaps 25–30 percent, the latter with one as low as 1 percent. It was *variola major* or varieties of similar deadliness that, for obvious reasons, had the greatest impact and which most often forced their way into historical records. If one were to compose a list of the dozen or so infections that have most undeniably affected the course of humanity, smallpox would have to be included.

Smallpox could spread via pox pus or scabs, but in the enormous majority of cases did so when the susceptible inhaled the virus exhaled by people sick with the disease. The distance crossed in transmission was seldom more than a few meters, but that was sufficient to enable the infection to spread quickly through closely packed populations. Long-range transmission was common, too, because the incubation period of the disease was about a dozen days, during which an infected but not yet actively ill individual could travel scores – and after the invention of railroads, steam ships and airplanes even thousands – of miles.

There never was a cure. Even the twentieth century's antibiotics had no more direct effect upon it than upon any other viral, as contrasted with bacterial, infection, though they did help enormously to prevent secondary infections.

After the incubation period the victim was struck down swiftly, even abruptly, by high fever and severe pains in the head, back and muscles. In the very worst cases, the story ended at this early stage with hemorrhages in the lungs and other organs. Most people lived on at least another two to five days when the characteristic rash appeared. Soon after that the pimples developed into full-scale pustules. In some sufferers these were so dense that they overlapped – this was called confluent smallpox – practically eliminating the skin, opening the way to all sorts of secondary infections and, in almost all instances, making death inevitable. For most of the afflicted the pustules were fewer, more widely spaced, and the chances of survival much better. If they survived the feverish crisis, their pustules dried and the scabs fell off a few weeks later. Pockmarks, lasting for a lifetime, were a common legacy

A coin to commemorate Elizabeth I's recovery from smallpox.

of the disease, ranging from the mild disfigurement of a George Washington to the ravaged faces of some, whose skin, in Herman Melville's words, was left 'like the complicated ribbed bed of a torrent, when the rushing waters have been dried up'.

Smallpox could not have existed in prehistoric times with the characteristics by which we identify it. Its virus had no host except humans, could not live long outside the human body, and either killed its hosts and died with them or stimulated their immune systems to raise up a strong and long-lasting immunity to the virus, completely eliminating it from the host, thereby blocking chances of future transmission. The sparse populations of hunter-gatherers could not have sustained the disease any more than a scattering of trees can sustain a forest fire.

Once it did appear, its communicability among and between dense populations guaranteed that most adults in such environments caught the disease while young and, if they survived, enjoyed lifetime immunity. In many regions transmission of the disease was limited to children as was the case with measles and mumps in most societies in the first half of this century. There are legions of exceptions, but it is a useful rule to think of smallpox as a disease of the children of civilization.

Where and when did it first appear? In the eastern hemisphere for certain. We know that because of the swiftness with which the disease spread among Amerindians after 1492

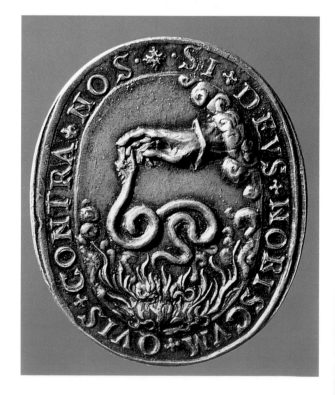

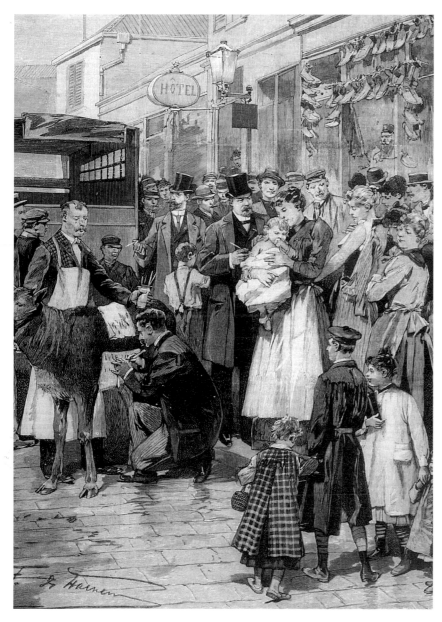

epidemics of pustular infection among the peoples of the ancient civilizations – for instance, those of the Roman Empire in the second and third centuries AD – but again we cannot be sure of their identity. It might have been smallpox, but it might have been measles, or even scarlet fever. Smallpox may have afflicted the Chinese by the fourth century, and almost certainly struck Japan in the 730s.

'Almost' becomes 'certainly' in the ninth century with the writing of *The Treatise on Smallpox and Measles* by Rhazes, a physician of Baghdad on the Tigris. He described clearly the differences between the two usually confused infections, and told his first readers what they no doubt already knew, that smallpox was common as a childhood disease in his part of the world. If so, considering the communicability of the disease, then it was probably endemic elsewhere in the strip of dense population that stretched from Morocco and Portugal to China. By this time it must have also been making epidemic excursions into the Eurasian steppe, northern Europe, and even sub-Saharan Africa. In those lands it would have struck people of all ages with brief but crushing effect, as a large percentage of the population would have been simultaneously laid low in each epidemic.

However, insofar as we can judge from the documents, smallpox was not an inevitably fatal disease in the period from Rhazes to the sixteenth century. The attitude in Europe, at least, was that smallpox was an unpleasant but survivable experience that children had to go through.

Smallpox first crossed the Atlantic in 1519 and had not just unpleasant but catastrophic effects in the Americas, playing a crucially important role in the European conquests of the great Amerindian empires. After their defeat, the Aztecs recorded that as they had prepared for the Spanish siege of their capital, Tenochtitlán, the disease struck and

'There was a great havoc. Very many died of it. They could not walk; they only lay in their resting places and beds. They could not move; they could not stir; they could not change position, nor lie on one side; nor face down, nor on their backs. And if they stirred, much did they cry out. Great was its destruction. Covered with pustules, very many people died of them.'

and among Australian Aborigines and Pacific islanders when they, in turn, were contacted by mainlanders and exposed to their infections. Smallpox probably first appeared among people with domesticated livestock, cattle and horses most likely, who suffer similar pox infections. Shepherds and their herds lived elbow-to-elbow, haunch-to-haunch and elbow-to-haunch, passing all kinds of parasites back and forth, micro and macro, intra and inter-species, creating an ideal situation for the development of new strains. An educated guess would give the birthplace of this infection as somewhere in or beside the great river civilizations of what are modern-day Iraq, Pakistan and Egypt.

The body of Pharaoh Ramses V, who died in 1157 BC, shows what may be smallpox pustules on the face, neck and shoulders. This may be our earliest evidence of the disease, but mummification and the passage of 3,000 years have rendered the diagnosis unsure. There were well-documented

FACING, LEFT: Georges Jacques Danton (1759–94) was badly scarred by smallpox as a child. When guillotined in 1794 he told the executioner to hold his head up high 'as the people would find it worthwhile'.

ABOVE LEFT: Taking blood from a calf, for the purposes of vaccination against smallpox. Paris street scene.

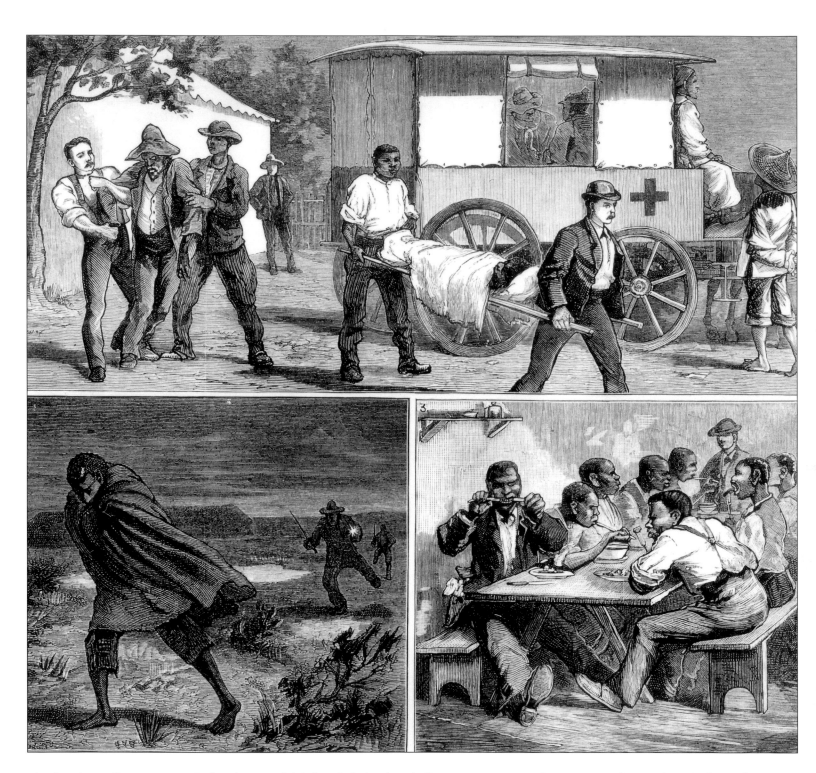

Sketches of a smallpox epidemic in Cape Town. Wood engraving.

Perhaps because of their long isolation Amerindians were genetically more susceptible to smallpox than Europeans, or perhaps this was the nature of every epidemic of the disease among what epidemiologists call a virgin soil population. The death rate of Iceland's entirely European population, visited in 1707 with smallpox for the first time in a generation, was over 25 percent, some say as high as a third. Perhaps the strain that crossed the Atlantic was not the mild one circulating in

Europe, but a more virulent one brought from Africa in the first years of the Atlantic slave trade. Or perhaps the smallpox virus coincidentally evolved into a deadlier strain for its own mysterious reasons.

Whatever the cause, while smallpox slaughtered the Amerindian peoples, it also began to kill European children in greater percentages than before. During the sixteenth, seventeenth and eighteenth centuries the disease, endemic in

Europe's ports and large cities and epidemic in the hinterlands, was one of the commonest of major infections and causes of death, especially for children. As the Black Death, the bubonic plague, retreated from its role as one of the most efficient controllers of population size, smallpox advanced to take its place.

Various efforts were made to control and cure the disease. Quarantine sometimes worked, though the infection, with its long incubation period, often found ways to spread anyway. All sorts of quackery were exercised – for instance, red curtains for the sickroom because of the reddish appearance of the pustuled sufferers – but to no avail. Curing smallpox was impossible. But was there a way to prevent people from getting the disease in the first place? Upper-class Europeans and their degree-laden physicians were unaware of it, but in some parts of Africa and Eurasia people had for a long time practiced a primitive sort of vaccination we call variolation. Smallpox contracted in the usual way by breathing in the virus often killed a fourth and even more of sufferers. But the great majority – 95, 98 and even 99 percent – of those who got the disease artificially, when the pus and scabs from the pocks of active cases were scratched into their skin – recovered! This miracle was first brought to the attention of western élites by an African slave of the Massachusetts Bay Colony's minister, Cotton Mather, and by Lady Mary Wortley Montagu, wife of the British ambassador in Constantinople, who learned of it there. Variolation was first tried out on a large scale during a smallpox epidemic in Boston, Massachusetts, in 1721. Fourteen percent of those who caught the disease the usual way died. Just under 2.5 percent of those who caught it via variolation died.

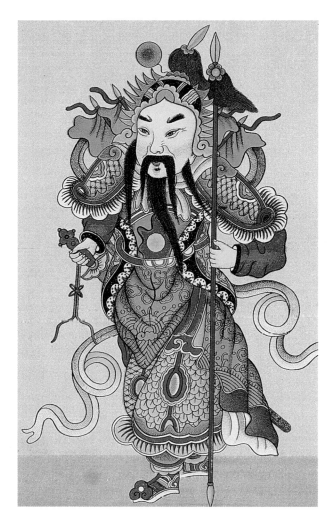

Yuo-hoa-long, the Chinese god of recovery from smallpox.

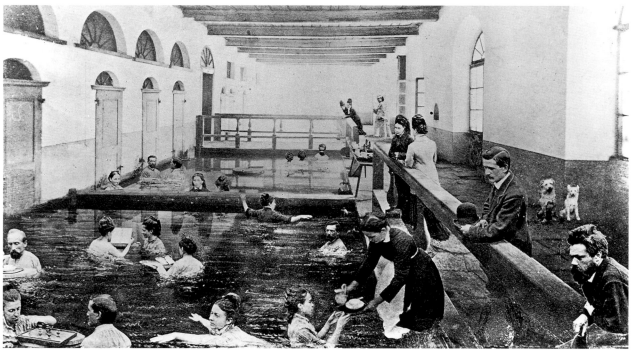

Baths at Hoeche in Valais, Switzerland, c. 1873. By the end of the century, the belief that baths were efficacious in curing smallpox had been replaced by vaccination.

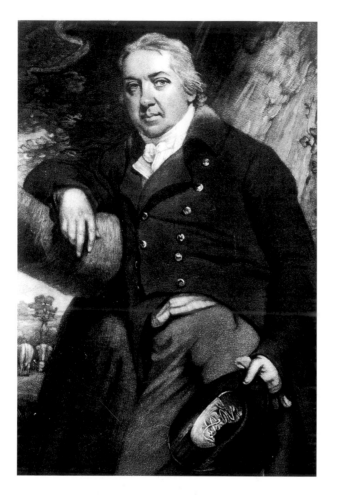

Edward Jenner (1749–1823), discoverer of vaccination.

The practice spread widely in western societies, especially after Louis XV of France died of smallpox in 1774, though by no means did it become universal. General George Washington, for instance, had his soldiers, many of whom were country folk who had never even seen the disease, variolated for fear that his army, barely able to survive encounters with the British Redcoats, might be decimated by an encounter with smallpox.

Some of the variolated died of the disease anyway. Some died from secondary infections they received along with smallpox via variolation. Many died in epidemics started unintentionally via variolation. The death rate of the variolated might be low, but that of people who caught the disease from them was still high. The true importance of variolation is not the number it saved in the eighteenth century, but the fact that it prepared the scientific and public minds for vaccination.

Toward the end of that century Edward Jenner, an English physician, noticed that variolation did not cause smallpox in some of his patients. These were individuals who had already had a mild disease, commonly called cowpox, caught from livestock, usually cattle. He inoculated people, including his son, who had never had smallpox, with cowpox matter, and found that they were immune to smallpox. The technique was the same as variolation, but the matter transferred came from a different source, so he called it 'vaccination', derived from the Latin word for cow.

In 1798 Jenner presented to the world the results of his discovery, one of the most important ever made in the field

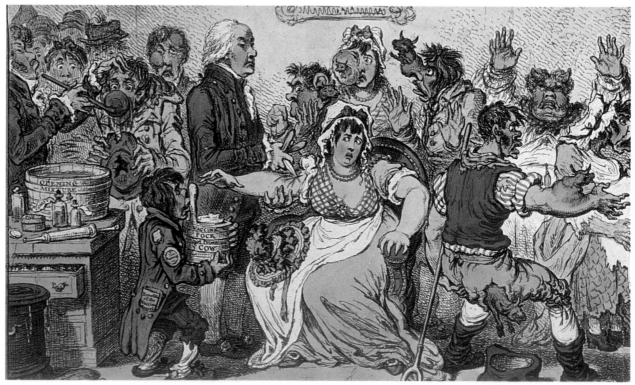

Coloured etching, 'The Cow-Pock – the wonderful effects of the new inoculation'. Not everyone could at first accept that vaccinations could work. By James Gillray, 1802.

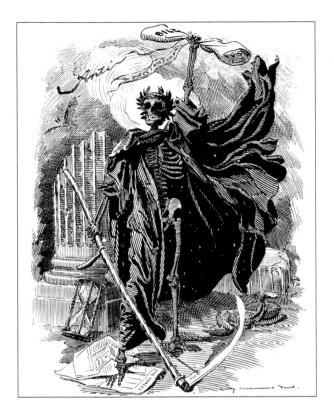

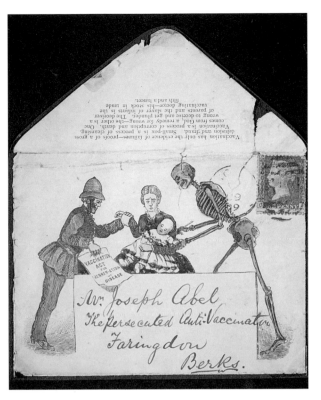

LEFT: *Anti-vaccination propaganda, 1899. The back of the envelope starts: 'Vaccination has only the evidence of failures ...'*
FAR LEFT: *'Triumph of De-Jenneration.' Punch cartoon, 30 July 1898. Death holds aloft the Vaccination bill, 'The Bill for the Encouragement of Smallpox'.*

of medicine: *An Inquiry into the Causes and Effects of Variolae Vaccinae, a Disease, Discovered in some of the Western Counties of England, particularly of Gloucestershire, and known by the Name of Cow Pox.* Three years later it was available in German, French, Spanish, Dutch, Italian and Latin. By 1801 more than 100,000 had been vaccinated in England, by 1811 more than 1.7 million in France, and so on around the world. In 1804 Don Francisco Xavier Balmis, backed by the Spanish monarchy, carried the practice of vaccination across the Atlantic to Spanish America, on to the Philippines and then back home in a therapeutic odyssey that lasted two years.

In England and Prussia the number of smallpox deaths fell to nearly zero by 1900, but vaccination was sporadic and far from universal outside Europe and North America. Scores of millions more fell ill with the disease of whom millions, usually the children, died. The appearance and spread of *variola minor*, with a death rate about as low as that of smallpox acquired via expert variolation, toward the end of the nineteenth century was a lagniappe, but smallpox, if no longer what Jenner called 'the most dreadful scourge of the human race', remained among the several most dreadful.

The difference between it and the others, malaria and tuberculosis for instance, was that humanity knew how to eliminate it completely, at least in theory. Vaccination produced lasting immunity. There were no animal reservoirs of the infection, and the virus was too fragile to last long outside the human body. Vaccinate everyone on earth, and the disease could be extinguished.

But did you have to vaccinate *everyone*, every last one of humanity's billions? No, fortunately. Locating every active case – an enormous task in itself – and then vaccinating everyone who had any contact with the patient would stop the disease. People beyond that endangered circle would not get it simply because it would not be available to be caught.

By 1972 there was no smallpox in South America. By 1974 none except in India, possibly the birthplace of the disease, and in the horn of Africa, Ethiopia and Somalia. The last case of normally contracted *V. major* occurred in Bangladesh in October 1975. The last case of *V. minor*, the final case of smallpox contracted in the usual way, was in Somalia in October 1977. The Global Commission for the Eradication of Smallpox waited two years for new cases to appear and then, in 1979, announced the complete eradication of the scourge – one of the greatest triumphs of scientific knowledge and public health practice in history.

BIBLIOGRAPHY

Behbehani, Abbas M. 1988. *The Smallpox Story in Words and Pictures.* Kansas City, Kansas.
Bowers, John Z. 1981. 'The Odyssey of Smallpox Vaccination', *Bulletin of the History of Medicine*, vol. 55, pp. 17–33.
Crosby, Alfred W. 1972. *The Columbian Exchange: Biological and Cultural Consequences of 1492.* Westport, Conn.
Dixon, D. W. 1962. *Smallpox.* London.
Henderson, Donald A. 1988. *Smallpox Eradication.* Geneva.
Hopkins, Donald R. 1983. *Princes and Peasants: Smallpox in History.* Chicago.

CHAPTER 12

MEASLES: THE RED MENACE

By Ann G. Carmichael

Of all the great epidemic diseases, measles has been the most underrated. Even in the dramatic virgin soil epidemics that rapidly reduced or eliminated indigenous populations of the western hemisphere, Australia and most of the Pacific islands, measles is accorded mere accomplice status. Westerners readily apprehend smallpox as a great killer – it is the 'usual suspect'. It is an effort for us to accept measles as a dread disease. Instead the unique vulnerabilities – often viewed as genetic frailties – of native populations outside Europe, Asia and Africa are blamed for measles mortality. These peoples are viewed as 'natural' victims.

There are two ways in which measles has acquired this domesticated, non-threatening profile. First, the virus that causes measles has evolved with primates and human global conquest, so measles accompanies the leading edge of 'civilization' in human history. Second, during the last 150 years measles in industrialized regions has been firmly attached to the public presence of children – to schools and orphanages and the various festivals associated with rites of passage from infancy through puberty. European societies, including their colonial possessions, became more child-conscious during this period, even as the overall proportion of children in society was decreasing. Measles came into focus because children did, too; measles belonged to the nursery.

The first great domestication of measles must have occurred in distant prehistory. In its nucleic sequences the measles virus is most closely related to the canine distemper virus and to bovine rinderpest. It requires but a small leap of the imagination to understand the emergence of a human variant of these with the domestication of animals. The measles that survives today infects only humans and monkeys.

This chameleon killer cannot survive if it fails to find new humans to infect, because once a host has survived the virus's assault, he is immune. From the virus's point of view – if a being 20 nanometers in diameter may be fondly portrayed as having a point of view – dead hosts and immune hosts are equally useless. The virus can make the necessary billions of copies of itself only when its host cannot yet target and kill the cells where measles has set up shop. To survive the evolutionary lottery measles has to find a susceptible host, replicate madly and then break away to a new home within ten to seventeen days. The efficient virus does this by passing to the next host *before* the first host gets sick, before the red rash betrays its maker, and by being mild enough so that people are perfectly able to travel and work before they and others recognize the illness. Measles evolved in great cities and the bustle that surrounded them; it needs a minimum host population size of around 250,000 in order to survive month after month, year after year.

It is possible that measles emerged many times, and some recent episodes illustrate how constant change and adaptation are in morbilliviruses (the genera to which measles belongs). In the late 1980s and early 1990s, seals worldwide, but especially in the north Atlantic, died of a similar kind of virus; lions in the Serengeti plain of east Africa were recently stricken with a distemper-like virus acquired from wild dogs near the nature preserve; a lone groomsman in Australia sickened from a measles-like virus acquired from a horse. Interspecies adaptation of morbilliviruses seems the rule; the human virus we know is very stable and varies little. Nevertheless there is no mild strain, no virulent strain: just measles.

Measles is demoted even in its ancient names. It has long been 'just' measles – a word from medieval terms for spots or excrescences, even on pork that has spoiled. The Latin term, *morbilli,* means 'little plague' and is the diminutive of *morbus,* plague. And it was long confused with diseases we deem deadlier: smallpox and scarlet fever. Historically it is surprising that for all its presumed antiquity there is no description of measles from Greco-Roman texts, nor from Chinese or Indian documents securely predating the last millennium. The earliest written account comes from the early tenth century, from the pen of a legendary Muslim physician, Rhazes. Attempting to differentiate smallpox from measles, Rhazes focused on predicting the outcomes of individual cases and on lessening suffering. Rhazes noted the

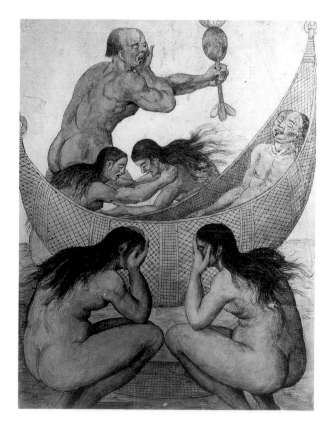

Native Brazilians mourning their dead. Mass death followed the Spanish conquest of the continent as the indigenous peoples were exposed for the first time to new diseases.

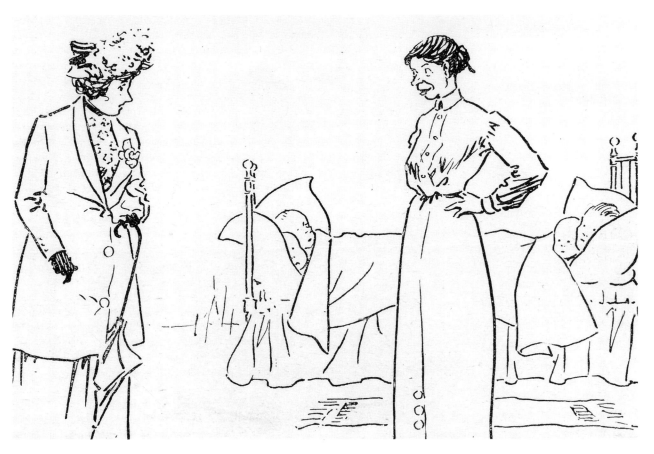

A London Mail *cartoon, 1915, gently ridicules a poor mother's protest to the district nurse: she has separated her infected children from the others by placing them at opposite ends of the available bed.*

depth of the redness, the location and quickness of pain, the pace of the breathing; he recommended procedures that he believed would help speed up the progression to a 'crisis', which served as gateway to recovery or to death.

A century later, another Muslim physician, the great Persian scientist known to the West as Avicenna, provided a theoretical context for the pathology and therapeutics of rash-producing diseases. Avicenna extrapolated from Galenic and Aristotelian biology that residual menstrual blood from the mother was incompletely 'cooked' or changed into the growing body's humors and solid parts. Fetal development, infancy and childhood provided ample opportunities to resolve or transform the residual menstrual blood, and the clinical appearance was a rash, a lobster-red one. Rashes could change in color, distribution, severity or appearance (for example, either pustular, flat or raised like sandpaper rashes might result) depending on the nature of the uncooked menstrual matter. But the longer the mother's menses resided in the offspring, the more dangerous the resultant disease. Rhazes and Avicenna thus provided an epidemiological theory: later onset of the rash in an individual's life predicted a more severe, more dangerous clinical course.

In the ninth and tenth centuries Islamic lands were much more populous than the predominantly rural, regionally isolationist Christian Europe. As the European population expanded in the twelfth and thirteenth centuries, however, first the Arabic texts and then the acknowledgment of disease

phenomena like measles were appropriated by western physicians. It is impossible to determine whether measles was imported from the Middle East or finally noticed by better prepared minds.

Increasing attention to human anatomy in the Renaissance, to reading the human body as a kind of text, facilitated further differentiation of rash-inducing diseases. In the sixteenth and seventeenth centuries, several well-published clinicians noted differences between measles and scarlet fever, not by focusing on skin blebs or predicting outcomes, but rather by observing the distribution of the rash on the body. Scarlet fever rarely affects the face, but the rashes of measles and smallpox become confluent there early in the illness. Instead of looking at which bodies were predisposed to measles, European physicians increasingly looked at what measles did to bodies.

Thomas Sydenham, a successful London physician of the late seventeenth century, produced a classic description of the ordinariness of measles. The contrast between Sydenham's detached clinical observation of disease phenomena in the bodies of young patients and the earlier account by Rhazes is striking. Rhazes began: 'Bodies that are lean, bilious, hot and dry, are more disposed to the Measles than to the Small Pox.' Sydenham began: 'The measles generally attack children. On the first day they have chills and shivers, and are hot and cold in turns.' Measles had become something one had, not a reflection of what one was.

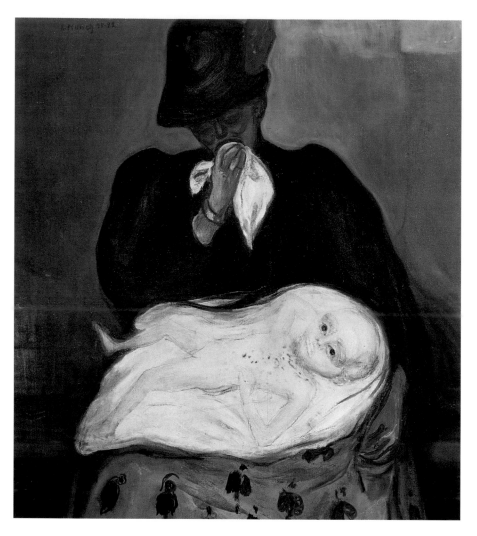

*'The Inheritance', by
Edvard Munch (1863–
1944).*

Though distinctive in its disease status, measles was not a problem which provoked public action until the nineteenth century, when European governments suddenly had to deal with unexpected, occasionally catastrophic, consequences of a measles epidemic in some remote settlement or colonial possession. While measles was clearly a part of the incidental disease background of early-modern health controls – it was routinely mentioned in most early cause-of-death registration systems – differentiating measles from many other miasms and contagions seemed hopeless and relatively unimportant wherever more feared, or more costly, diseases threatened (e.g., smallpox, plague, malaria, phthisis, yellow fever and, by 1832, Asiatic cholera). But during a phase sometimes described as the 'expansion' period of measles in human history, the routine behavior of measles virus, acting alone, finally became noticeable.

A 26-year-old medical graduate of the University of Copenhagen, Peter Ludwig Panum, harvested most of the credit for unmasking the measles' *modus operandi*. In 1846 the Danish government dispatched a medical team to give aid during an explosive measles epidemic in the Faeroes, an archipelago of eighteen islands then restricted to exclusive trade and commerce with Denmark. Panum and a colleague, Manicus, arrived two months into a severe epidemic of measles, by which time the fourth or fifth 'generation' of measles victims were just becoming ill. (The first victim fell ill in late March. His contacts formed the second generation, and so on until early June, when Panum and Manicus arrived.) Most of their work became a retrospective epidemiological investigation rather than a rescue mission. The epidemic was over by July, at which point roughly 6,100 of the 7,864 Faeroese islanders had been stricken with the measles.

Several things made this study classic and elegant. The victims themselves could provide an accurate account of where they went, who they saw and when, for the geographical isolation of the Faeroes made visits and social occasions memorable. From interviews Panum (who gets almost all of the credit because he wrote the report) could demonstrate that people contracted measles from those who were in the 'prodromal' or 'catarrhal' stage of the disease. Before the distinctive measles rash appeared, victims seemed to be catching a bad cold or flu. They had watery eyes, nasal congestion, perhaps a cough and sore throat – symptoms far too commonplace to warrant quarantine. There had been a severe epidemic of measles in 1781, sixty-five years previously, and in 1846 the Faeroese quickly quarantined those who broke out in a rash. But Panum was now able to prove that by the time the rash appeared quarantine was too late.

Panum also suggested that the 'efflorescence' – the flowering of a rash on the skin – contained no 'morbific matter' that passed the disease. The measles was a contagion, but the contagion was not lodged in the rash, which appeared on day fourteen. Finally, Panum discovered that those who lived through the 1781 epidemic did not contract measles in 1846; lifelong immunity to the disease upon recovery was possible. In subsequent epidemics in the Faeroes during the later nineteenth century, the ambiguous cases among Panum's observations were clarified: only those individuals who were more than eighteen months old when they contracted measles were fully immune the next time they were exposed.

Panum and Manicus did not clearly understand how deadly measles could be, however. The Faeroes were not quite virgin soil to the measles virus; that is, because some members of the population had been exposed to measles before, not everyone was susceptible. Historically, the period of 'expansion' is associated with virgin soil epidemics, the worst of which were probably those suffered by Amerindians before European immigrants could help or even record the mortality.

Virgin soil epidemics of acute infectious diseases cause tremendous loss of life because many fall ill at the same time. The specific causes of the increased mortality, however, are not fully attributable to the pathological effects of the particular infectious agent. If a large group of people, such as the millions occupying central Mexico at the time of the early Spanish conquistadors, are infected within the same couple of months, the adults may be too ill to attend to the babies' normal hygienic and nutritional needs. The old will be at risk because they have less ability to withstand the complications, such as dehydration, pneumonia and gastrointestinal disease. Measles and most viral infections are, however, oddly stressful to young adults, the population's strongest and healthiest in normal circumstances. Even outside virgin soil circumstances, measles and smallpox are more severe if the patient has reached adulthood. Thus the extra recovery time needed for young adult providers quickly unravels the entire population's usual methods of weathering the crisis. Food, clean water, personal hygiene, even the resolve to live, are elusive or absent resources of the community.

In Alaska, during the gold rush of 1900, communities were hit by influenza and measles; those that were struck by both at once were devastated. Those that had any access at all to healthy care-givers fared better than those who had not. Tiny villages, especially isolated settlements far from population centers, were nearly exterminated.

The Epidemiological Society in London came to appreciate the severity of measles only after it was introduced into the Fiji Islands in 1875. The Fiji Islands had attracted expanding British colonial interests in Australia and New South Wales, as well as the missionary zeal of migratory Wesleyans. The approximate native population was 150,000. Early in 1875 the governor of New South Wales invited King Cakobau, Fiji's most powerful chieftain, to visit, returning the king and his two sons to Levuka by way of HMS *Dido*. The king was ill but recovering from measles upon arrival; his sons were quite sick. All had contracted the disease during the twenty-two-day voyage.

Although the news of a sick king was communicated to shore before docking, the *Dido* did not fly the yellow flag of quarantine, and no one was prevented from disembarking. Cakobau summoned many other chiefs to his palace, and at the end of January met sixty-nine chieftains and their entourages (*c.* 500 people in all), together with some crew members from the *Dido* and administrators from the Admiralty. Two other British ships arrived from Sydney at the same time, both conveying children ill with measles and their anxious mothers.

The surviving islanders attributed the subsequent disaster to poison, treachery or bewitchment. A report was made to the London Epidemiological Society: 'The attacks are so sudden and complete that every soul in a village will be down at once; and no one will be able to procure food, or if obtainable, to cook it for themselves or others. The people have died from exhaustion and starvation in the midst of plenty.' Mortality was estimated at 26 percent – 'not less than 40,000', according to the Fiji colonial governor – making the epidemic as severe as most European plagues.

Measles had had an unequivocal, though punctuated, historical presence in Japan since the Middle Ages, but epidemics occurred at relatively distant and irregular intervals. Measles was both rare and clearly disseminated from Nagasaki, the only port open to foreign trade, so measles was a feared disease in Japan.

Meanwhile in most European cities at the end of the nineteenth century – London is an especially well-documented, well-studied example – measles was curiously resilient at a time when other infectious diseases were receding. Mandatory nationwide notification of scarlet fever by 1889 may have prompted an increase in reports of children with measles, but measles itself did not carry the

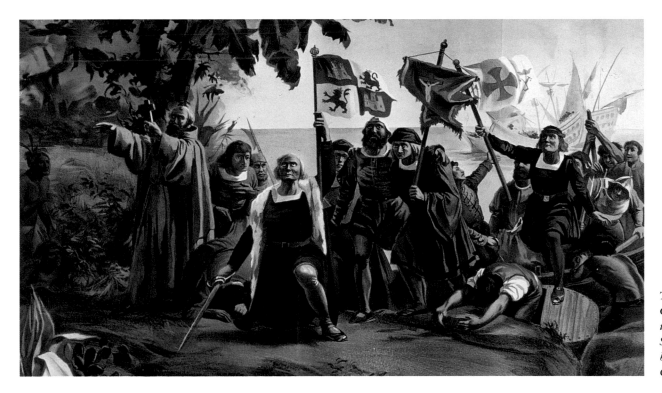

The first landing of Columbus on the shores of the New World at San Salvador, 12 October 1492, by D. Puebla, published by Currier and Ives.

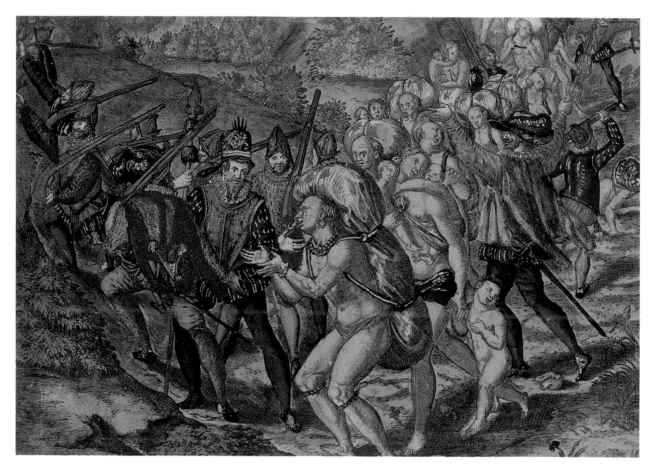

same efforts at control. But the plain fact emerging from more intensive health surveillance was that significant numbers of young children died or suffered long illnesses precipitated by a bout of measles.

Measles was clearly associated with poverty. But what was it that insured higher death rates among destitute children? Later twentieth-century clinical and epidemiological studies of measles in west Africa suggest that both malnutrition (protein calorie deprivation as well as generalized caloric deficiency) and crowding exacerbate measles infection. Malnourished toddlers develop a deep red-brown, confluent measles rash, followed by severe respiratory and gastrointestinal complications. Many children crowded together, either in institutions or individual households, may, according to some investigators, suffer severe cases of measles simply because they experience a heavy exposure or 'viral load'. Poor children are often exposed as well to tuberculosis and other chronic infections, helping to insure the high measles death rates.

Quite suddenly, in the mid-1910s, in the middle of World War I, mortality began to plummet in the United Kingdom. Treatment had not suddenly improved, but epidemic disease surveillance intensified and, more importantly, the War Office devoted resources to ameliorating the material and nutritional conditions of

working mothers. The improvement has been characterized as one leading from destitution to mere deprivation.

The War Office was fighting measles because it was a military problem, following the outbreak of epidemics in military camps. We know that the incidence and prevalence of measles reached alarming proportions, and often accompanied mobilization. Soldiers from cities had usually been exposed to measles in childhood, but farm-boys of many nations were stricken even on transport trains to the training barracks. The health costs of measles were learned early in the war, especially at the Allies' defeat at Gallipoli. Troops were amassed for the assault in crowded encampments near Cairo, allowing rapid spread of the virus; infected soldiers marched blithely into battle.

First continental, then intercontinental warfare consolidated measles experience globally, just as colonization had done. During the American Civil War of the 1860s, measles infection accounted for 98,817 cases and 2,367 deaths among four million enlisted men. These data come from only the more urbanized, industrialized Union army, for most routine records of the Confederate operations were destroyed. Losses attributed to measles were far heavier in the Confederate army. This regional differentiation continued through US mobilizations in the Spanish–American war and again in World War I, vividly illustrating that early childhood exposure to measles, if in a privileged economic environment, was the best available protection.

Rather than the 'expansion' of measles into remote non-measly islands, then, the military exploits of western nations before 1950 served to redefine measles as a domestic menace, and to focus attention on the problems of differential mortality across race, class and region, and to view the control of measles as important to national security.

The final, ongoing stage of measles history marks a retreat. Vaccination against measles significantly accelerated its decline. Vaccines for measles initially followed the apparent success of the Salk polio vaccine, and killed virus vaccines became available in the early 1960s. The American virologist Jonas Salk had decided that it was too risky to use a live polio virus vaccine, though he knew that all successful viral vaccines (including Edward Jenner's cowpox and Louis Pasteur's rabies vaccines) used weakened (or 'attenuated') strains of a live virus. Salk created a killed virus vaccine, and in 1954 proved that it immunized against polio. Meanwhile, virologist Albert Sabin produced a live, attenuated, polio vaccine, the one we use today.

Salk's success led to the hope of a killed, thus 'safe', measles vaccine, which initially sold better than the live virus vaccine. By the early 1970s, however, cases of 'atypical' measles occurred among those people given killed vaccine. Atypical measles was true measles, but difficult to recognize because the rash pattern was unusual.

Measles, being an exclusively human infection, could be eradicated by much the same methods that the World Health Organization used to defeat smallpox. Instead, pediatricians and general practitioners are left explaining to well-educated parents that protection from this infection is worth the baby's discomfort. On the global front, annual measles mortality has recently been estimated at two million deaths. Measles is still very much at home.

BIBLIOGRAPHY

Cliff, Andres, Haggett, Peter and Smallman-RaynorMatthew . 1993. *Measles: An Historical Geography of a Major Human Viral Disease.* London.

Corney, Bolton Glanville. 1883–4. 'The behaviour of certain epidemic diseases in natives of Polynesia with special reference to Fiji', *Transactions of the Epidemiological Society of London*, new series, 3, pp. 7694.

Hardy, Anne. 1993. *The Epidemic Streets: Infectious Disease and the Rise of Preventive Medicine, 1856–1900*, pp. 28–55. Oxford.

Jannetta, Ann Bowman. 1987. *Epidemics and Mortality in Early Modern Japan.* Princeton.

Major, Ralph H. 1965. *Classic Descriptions of Disease* (3rd edn). Springfield, Illinois

Panum, Peter Ludwig. 1939. 'Observations made during the epidemic of measles in the Faeroe Islands in the year 1846', *Medical Classics 3*, pp. 803–86.

Wolfe, Robert J. 1982. 'Alaska's great sickness, 1900: an epidemic of measles and influenza in a virgin soil population', *Proceedings of the American Philosophical Society 126*, pp. 911–21.

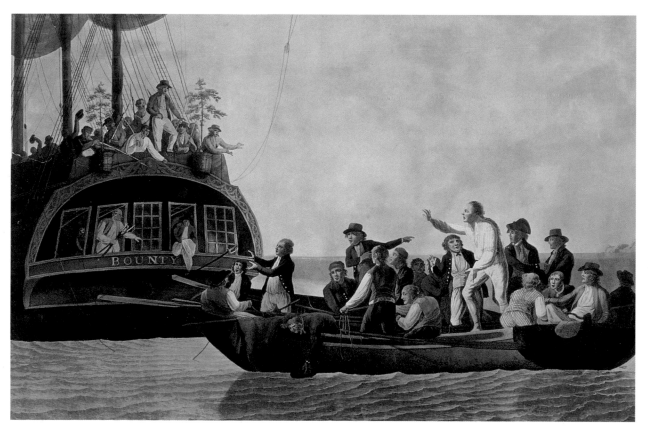

Mutiny on the Bounty, *1789. Captain Bligh was sent by the Admiralty to bring back breadfruit (seen in this picture) to improve nutrition in the West Indies. However, this scientific expedition brought new diseases into virgin territory. Engraving by Robert Dodd, 1789.*

CHAPTER 13

YELLOW FEVER: THE YELLOW JACK

By Margaret Humphreys

Yellow fever may well be an ancient disease, for it is so mild when at home, although nasty while traveling. At home, in the jungles of Africa and America, it lives quietly, infecting a cycle of mosquitoes and monkeys without making much of a fuss. Children living in the area meet the pathogen as part of the normal set of non-lethal childhood diseases, and thus acquire immunity. Undisturbed, this ecological pattern represents what would be expected of a mature prey/predator interaction, with the germ and its hosts in equilibrium. This was probably true for eons in Africa; with the transport of yellow fever to the New World, it came to be the case in the American tropics, probably by the nineteenth century.

Yet this was the disease that brought terror to the hearts of Euro-Americans in the eighteenth and nineteenth centuries. It emerged as a major source of epidemics, at first in the port cities of western Africa, then on the slave ships, and finally in the Caribbean, due to the invasion of its African habitat by slavers and other colonial despoilers. Unlike malaria, which could easily travel in chronically infected bodies, yellow fever had a much harder time making the Atlantic passage. Its cycle depends on an *aedes* mosquito biting an infected person, or monkey, then surviving for the time it takes the yellow fever virus to mature inside the insect, and finally finding a new, non-immune human to bite. The disease runs its course in seven to ten days, so there is only a short time for the sick person to offer up the virus to a new mosquito host. During a ten- to twelve-week voyage, this sequence would have to be maintained over several cycles of infection. And if the disease killed or made immune all the humans on board before the ship arrived at its next port, it would die out. Hence it is not surprising that it was not until 1647 that yellow fever successfully jumped the Atlantic, although the African slave trade had been underway for close to a century and a half.

There is controversy about this account. It has been argued that yellow fever originated in the American jungle, and from there traveled to ports on the Atlantic coast. Supporters of this view cite the fact that the disease first appears in accounts about the New World, and only later in descriptions of Africa. The strongest rebuttal to this claim lies in the evidence of innate immunity in both humans and monkeys of the respective continents. Both South American natives and the monkeys of the American tropics are very susceptible to yellow fever, while their counterparts in Africa have relative immunity. This may in fact explain why yellow fever was so 'invisible' in Africa – it did not become a terrifying disease until the Europeans arrived to both fall victim to it and report its ravages.

Yellow fever did not creep quietly into port; its dramatic symptoms and rapid mortality made it a loud and unmistakable visitor. Yellow fever is caused by a flavivirus, and is related to dengue and other Group B viruses. It mainly attacks the liver, bringing on that common symptom of hepatic failure, yellow jaundice. Since the liver produces components necessary for blood to clot, liver failure is often accompanied by bleeding. And the victim bleeds everywhere – from the nose, mouth, stomach, rectum and any open skin lesions. Blood in the stomach is turned black by gastric acid, and when vomited has the appearance of coffee grounds. This led to the Spanish name for the disease, *vomito negro*, and became as dramatic a sign of the presence of yellow fever as the bloodstained handkerchief was for tuberculosis. Other symptoms add to the patient's misery: high fever, palpitations, delirium, severe aching of the body and exhaustion. Kidney failure frequently intervenes in terminal cases. In a week or ten days it is over, with the patient either dead or convalescent (and subsequently immune).

The experience of watching a loved one die of yellow fever is terrible to imagine, as a letter written in 1897 which could as easily have served for any of the earlier epidemics vividly portrays. 'Lucille died at ten o'clock Tuesday night, after such suffering as I hope never again to witness,' wrote one man living in Memphis. He nursed this teenager, probably his niece, through an awful few days.

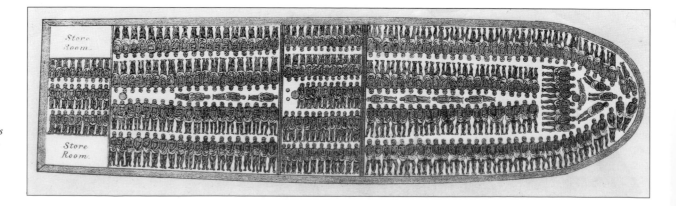

Diagram of a slave ship. The lower deck had slaves 'packed tight in the most inhuman way unable to breathe,' one physician observed.

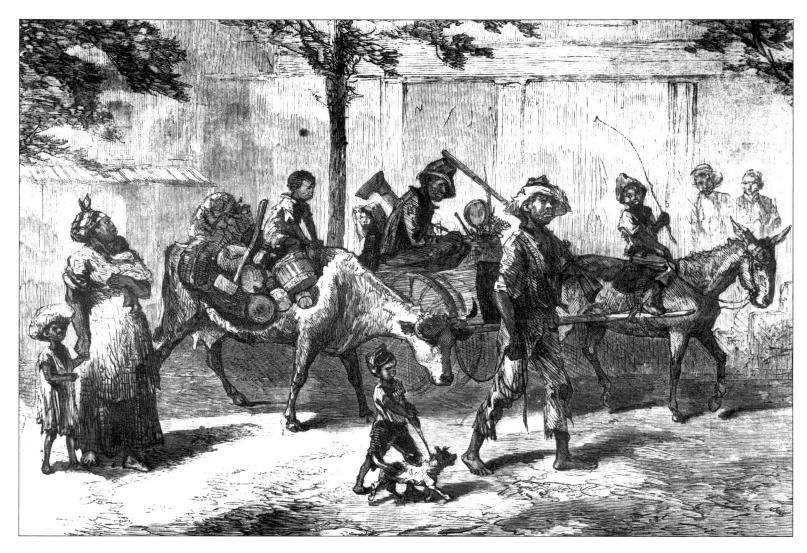

'Once or twice my nerve almost failed me, but I managed to stay. The poor girl's screams might be heard for a half a square and at times I had to exert my utmost strength to hold her in bed. Jaundice was marked, the skin being a bright yellow hue: tongue and lips dark, cracked and blood oozing from the mouth and nose. To me the most terrible and terrifying feature was the "black vomit" which I never before witnessed. By Tuesday evening it was as black as ink and would be ejected with terrific force. I had my face and hands spattered but had to stand by and hold her. Well it is too terrible to write any more about it.'

It is not surprising that panic and flight were common responses to exposure to such suffering.

One commanding aspect of the disease was its mortality. Modern estimates cite typical mortality rates of around 10 percent (that is, for every ten people who become ill, one will die of the disease). However, chroniclers of epidemics in the eighteenth and nineteenth centuries often put the figure much higher, at times as high as 70 percent. Both assessments may reflect reality. A major problem in estimating mortality rates is in determining how many people have been stricken with the disease. If the mildly ill are not counted, then the reported mortality rate will be inaccurately high, since those who are severely ill are also the most likely to die. Cases in children and in some people of African descent may be particularly invisible, skewing the data. It can be even more confusing when a large part of the population flees an epidemic. Then the number of people exposed in a town is unknown, and the proportion of the dead and dying who remain may assume an even greater impact. What is certain is that yellow fever caused great destruction wherever it found masses of non-immune adults, killing as it did with such gruesome symptoms.

Yellow fever was known as one of the 'seasoning' diseases in towns it visited frequently. Since established residents were immune from prior bouts of the disease, it was the newcomer who fueled the epidemic, giving rise to the name 'stranger's disease'. Many did not survive this initiation ritual, and this did much to minimize immigrant movement into subtropical port cities, which were viewed as more dangerous and diseased than their northern counterparts. Indeed, the Irish immigrants who chose New Orleans in the 1840s, for example, did much to feed

African-Americans on their way to resettle in Kansas in 1879, leaving behind the poverty and panic of yellow fever. Drawing by Sol Ettinge, Jr.

New Orleans Levee, 1884, the point where bananas, coffee and yellow fever frequently entered the United States, and left for the hinterland. Lithograph by Currier and Ives.

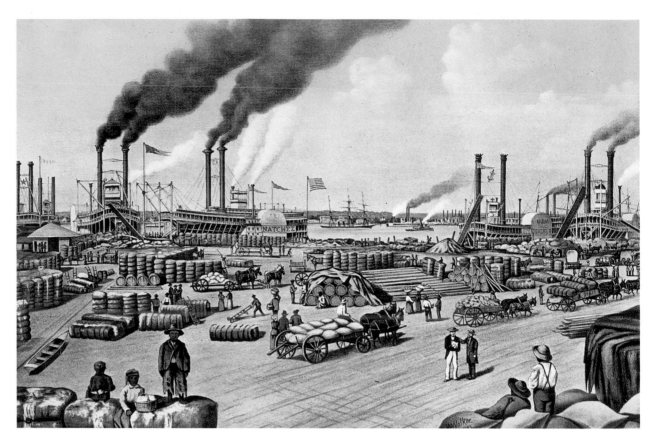

the flaming epidemics of yellow fever there in the 1850s. In fact, some southerners argued that the region wouldn't be diseased at all if these strangers would just stay out. Yellow fever limited population growth significantly wherever epidemics recurred.

After its first appearance in Barbados in 1647, yellow fever spread throughout the port cities of the American coast. First seen in St Kitts, Guadalupe, Cuba and the Yucatan Peninsula, by the eighteenth century it ranged from Brazil in the south as far north as Boston and New York in the English colonies. Europe was not spared either. Although epidemics there were less common than in the Americas, the port cities of Lisbon and Barcelona on the Iberian Peninsula, St Nazaire in France, and even Swansea in Wales were affected well into the nineteenth century.

Nothing in Europe compares to the impact that yellow fever had on Caribbean history, however. Along with malaria it was a principal force in making the islands inhospitable to Europeans. Like the western shores of Africa, the Caribbean Islands frequently became a 'white man's grave'. In 1655, for example, France sent 1,500 soldiers to conquer St Lucia; only eighty-nine survived the onslaught of yellow fever that met their arrival. When in 1741 Admiral Edward Vernon led 19,000 men of European descent in an attack on Cartagena, he lost half of his force to yellow fever. The disease also had a key role in the tempestuous last decade of the eighteenth century, when yellow fever and revolution swept through the Caribbean. The impact on North American communities was equally

significant. Florida lost so much of its population from yellow fever epidemics in the third and fourth decades of the nineteenth century that statehood was delayed. Memphis, in Tennessee, was nearly abandoned as uninhabitable after successive epidemics in 1878 and 1879, when the city lost its charter due to unpayable debts, and the large and affluent German immigrant population abandoned it for the healthier environs of St Louis.

Communities did not remain passive in the face of this dire threat. The association with ships coming from the tropics was quickly recognized, and vessels carrying pestilence were required to observe quarantines, and to fly a yellow warning flag, or jack. 'Yellow jack' became another nickname for the disease. Quarantine had emerged as a public health measure in the Middle Ages, when ships thought to be carrying bubonic plague were purified by forty days' isolation. Forty days was a traditional Judeo-Christian time of renewal and penance, from the forty days of Noah's flood to Christ's time in the wilderness, to the forty days of Lent. But forty days was a long time, especially if the ship in question bore perishable tropical goods such as bananas. Quarantines were fiercely opposed by commercial interests, and also frequently failed, since the mosquito could alight even when the crew could not.

Wherever it appeared yellow fever spurred public debate. Such a devastating illness demanded community response: something had to be done. Throughout the nineteenth century physicians in affected port cities debated how to subdue the disease, although until 1900 no accurate knowledge about its transmission was available. One side argued for strict quarantines to keep the disease, seen as a foreign invader, out. They based this on the idea that yellow fever was contagious, which might be hard to believe, since at times the disease jumped block to block between strangers. We can now explain this by having a mosquito fly out one window and into another, but the concept of person-to-person contagion couldn't be proven against yellow fever, because it did not happen. Still epidemics did seem to depend on the arrival from a yellow fever source of some sort of carrier, ship or person.

The other side of this debate believed that the roots of yellow fever lay in the filthy streets of the cities, acted on by the hot, humid climate of the summer months. The disease spontaneously generated, they argued, in the fetid air arising from rotting animals and human wastes. Cleaning the streets was the way to keep the sickness at bay. This could explain why a neighborhood could be struck by yellow fever even when the victims did not directly know one another, and also accorded with the disease's preference for the summer months (when, as we now know, the mosquito is most active). Still, there appeared to be seasons when all the causes were present, and there was no yellow fever. In New Orleans a physician made this point after a summer free of yellow fever: 'What a quandary the yellow fever wizards must be in!' he exclaimed. 'We have heat and moisture, dead dogs, cats, chickens, etc., all over the streets, and plenty of hungry doctors; yet Yellow Jack will not come.' He asked the key question, 'How does the present differ from some of the past, in regard to the *peculiar* conditions?'

From about the mid-nineteenth century physicians began to address the question of the cause of yellow fever in a new way.

Combining the two contending theories, they argued that a yellow fever 'seed' of some sort was transmitted from a city infected with the disease. It would take hold in a new site only if the 'soil' there was hospitable, namely if the environment was filthy enough to sponsor the growth of the seed into a full-blown epidemic. Thus both sanitation and quarantine were useful in keeping yellow fever out. The establishment of the germ theory in the last half of the nineteenth century changed everything. Now the search was on to find the yellow fever germ, which researchers assumed would be a bacterium like those which caused tuberculosis, cholera or pneumonia. In fact, though yellow fever bacteria were 'discovered' several times, it was always found that they were not the primary cause of the disease but merely germs which were secondary invaders in the ravaged body.

In 1899 Walter Reed, one of the most famous of American physicians, headed a commission sent by the Surgeon General to newly conquered Cuba in search of the cause of yellow fever. Reed and his colleagues first explored a bacterium proposed by an Italian researcher, Giuseppe Sanarelli. After dismissing this germ, which was the causative agent of hog cholera, Reed's group decided to test the hypothesis that the yellow fever germ, whatever it was, was carried by mosquitoes. Much historical debate has gone into the chronology on this issue. The dominant view is that Reed acquired the idea from the British army physician Ronald Ross, whose research on malaria and mosquitoes had appeared in 1897, since Reed saw that malaria and yellow fever seemed to occur in similar times and places. Others point to Carlos Finlay, a Cuban physician, who had proposed the mosquito transmission of yellow fever in the

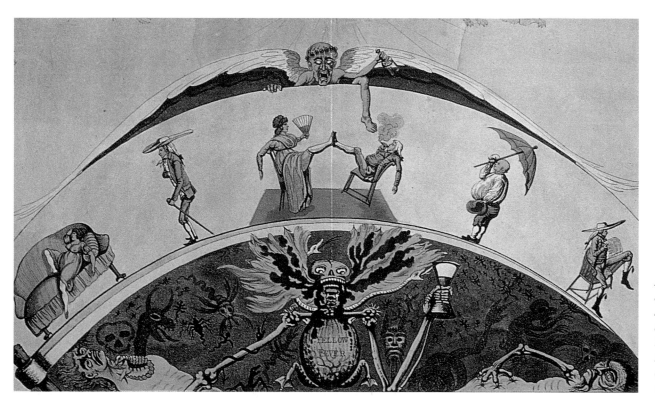

A parodic cosmology diagram showing opposing aspects of the life of colonialists in Jamaica – languorous noons and the hells of yellow fever. (Colored aquatint by A. J. 1800.)

1880s. It is hard to find a direct causal link between Finlay's ideas and Reed's, though, and Finlay had trouble demonstrating his argument because he focused on the wrong species of mosquito. He further clouded the issue by arguing for yet another false bacterial agent. In any event, there is no doubt that Walter Reed's group of researchers were the first to convince the world that yellow fever is spread by mosquitoes, and that, accordingly, controlling mosquitoes would lead to the control of the disease.

The Reed Commission's experimental plan was fairly simple. One group of volunteer soldiers was placed in a screened house. There they lived amid the filthy blankets and clothing of yellow fever patients, materials covered with vomit and other bodily wastes. If the germ of yellow fever lived anywhere, surely it was here. A second cohort of soldiers likewise inhabited a screened cottage but their living arrangements were pristine. All that happened to them was that they were exposed to mosquitoes that had bitten yellow fever patients. The results are well known. The soldiers living amid the sick bed effluvia were miserable but stayed healthy; their mosquito-bitten counterparts came down with yellow fever.

Not only did the Reed Commission establish the connection between mosquitoes and yellow fever, they also determined that the disease was caused by a virus. By 1900 medical researchers had realized that there were disease-causing agents smaller than bacteria, so small that they passed through pores in a filter that would have blocked any known bacterium. When the infectious serum of yellow fever patients was passed through such a filter, it retained its potency. Twenty years of searching for the yellow fever germ finally ended with the recognition that no one was going to find it with an ordinary microscope. During the 1930s researchers funded by the Rockefeller Foundation used this knowledge to create the first effective yellow fever vaccine.

Twentieth-century yellow fever battles were waged with these new weapons. William Crawford Gorgas was the first to show that controlling the mosquito would lead to controlling epidemics. First in Havana, and then in the famous case of the Panama Canal, he reduced the mosquito population through drainage, oiling breeding sites, and killing adult mosquitoes wherever they were found. He also focused on separating the viral reservoir (the yellow fever patient) from the mosquito, by screening the sick room, and burning the insecticide pyrethrum to kill any mosquitoes remaining in it. These methods of mosquito control were supplemented later in the century by arsenic larvicides, and then DDT, which killed adult mosquitoes very effectively. Combined with the vaccine, these tools caused the retreat of yellow fever back to its jungle home, where it persists, breaking out occasionally into tropical cities.

Cocoa plantation in the Isle of Grenada.

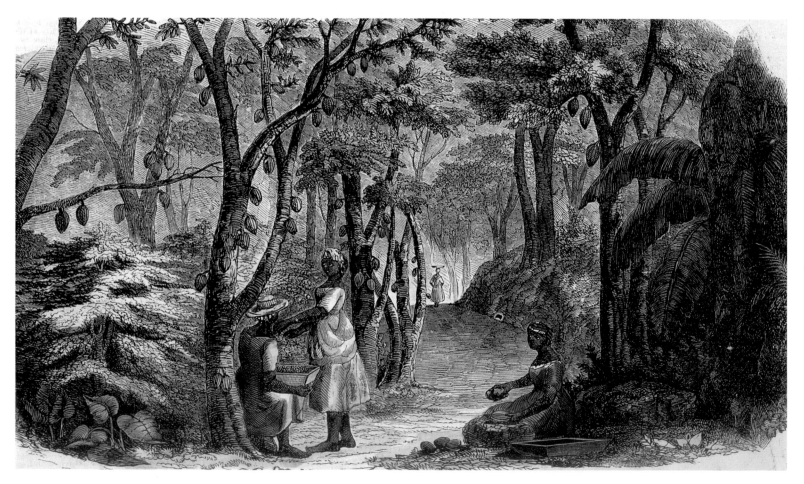

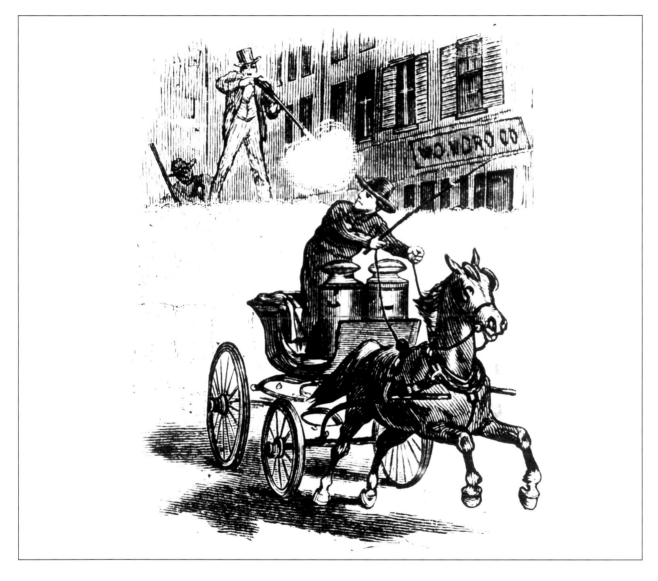

A milkman is shot while trying to cross yellow fever quarantine line in New Orleans. (Engraving, 1878.)

Questions about yellow fever remain. The major one concerns the fact that it has never invaded Asia, although abundant mosquitoes and suitable tropical environments certainly exist there. It is possible that inherited innate protection against yellow fever shields Asian populations; another theory holds that other infections, such as encephalitis, occupy the ecological niche of yellow fever, denying it a foothold. This puzzle is all the more intriguing because of a recent Asian import to the United States, the tiger mosquito, *aedes albopictus*, which appears perfectly capable of spreading yellow fever and its cousin, dengue fever. It is not at all clear why this mosquito is an effective vector on one continent and not on another.

Yellow fever serves as an early example of an 'emerging disease' and as a warning against the disruption of tropical habitats. In its jungle form the disease is not particularly threatening, and where it exists in equilibrium with a stable society, it causes only a minor childhood disease. Developed countries that disrupt such a balance do so at their peril.

In many ways it is fair to say that yellow fever is the price that Europeans and their progeny paid for the sin of slavery; certainly without the slave trade it is hard to imagine that the disease would have escaped very effectively from its jungle home.

BIBLIOGRAPHY
Coleman, William. 1987. *Yellow Fever in the North.* Madison, Wisconsin.
Cooper, Donald B. and Kenneth F. Kiple. 1993. 'Yellow Fever', in Kenneth F. Kiple (ed.), *The Cambridge World History of Human Disease Cambridge,* England and New York.
Curtin, Philip D. 1989. *Death by Migration: Europe's Encounter with the Tropical World in the Nineteenth Century.* Cambridge, England.
Humphreys, Margaret. 1992. *Yellow Fever and the South.* East Brunswick, New Jersey.
Monath, Thomas P. 1991. 'Yellow Fever: Victor, Victoria? Conqueror, Conquest? Epidemics and Research in the Last Forty Years and Prospects for the Future', *American Journal of Tropical Hygiene* 45, pp. 1–43.

M ost Americans and Europeans living in their own countries have lost their fear of mosquitoes. These pesky creatures may ruin a summer supper party on the veranda, or raise unsightly welts, but most members of the population do not respond to mosquito bites with significant concern for their health. This is a phenomenon of the modern era, for only in the last half century have Europe and North America been free of malaria, and yellow fever caused major damage in the United States as late as 1905. Although both these diseases continue to plague tropical areas, neither is a serious threat to the developed world today. A less well-known infection, dengue, is. Particularly spurred by the population explosion of its vector, the *Aedes* mosquito family, dengue may well become a major public health problem in the United States in coming years, and also threatens southern Europe. It is a burgeoning problem throughout the tropics, and there is little hope for its control in the foreseeable future. Although not usually fatal, this disease causes significant illness, destroys worker or soldier effectiveness, inhibits tourism, and does endanger the lives of some patients, especially children.

Dengue is caused by a virus in the flavivirus family, which includes the causative agent of yellow fever. There are four subtypes of dengue virus, and immunity to the disease comes only after the patient has had all four subtypes (called serotypes, and numbered Den 1–4). This complex immunity makes the creation of an effective vaccine particularly difficult. Like yellow fever, the virus is carried by mosquitoes of the *Aedes* family. The principal vector is *Aedes aegypti*, but in recent decades *Aedes albopictus* and other relatives have been implicated as well. In the past several years *Aedes albopictus*, known familiarly as the tiger mosquito, has colonized significant portions of the American South, making a massive pest of itself and setting the stage for the rapid spread of the dengue virus sometime in the future. *Aedes* species are urban dwellers, with preference for laying their eggs on the fresh water collected in water barrels, cisterns, drains, flower pots, tires or forgotten buckets.

The female mosquito is the disease transmitter, for it is she who requires blood meals to nourish her eggs. The dengue virus spends eight to eleven days inside the mosquito, replicating and moving to the salivary glands in preparation for the next time the mosquito finds a victim to feed on. The virus does not harm the mosquito, and she will remain infective for her lifetime, making multiple new cases possible from a single insect. After an incubation period in the human host of two to seven days – it varies with different dengue strains – there is an abrupt onset of clinical symptoms.

The distress caused by dengue is well encapsulated in its common name of 'breakbone fever'. The patient's first symptoms are frontal headache, sudden onset of fever, and muscle aches everywhere, especially in the lower back. Movement of the eyes can be particularly painful, described by patients as a deep soreness. Joint pains, vomiting, swollen lymph glands and a rash are all common, and follow over the next three to seven days. Patients are often apathetic and depressed, and may complain of disturbing dreams. One characteristic of dengue is that the fever will decline midcourse, and then spike for a couple of days at the end, producing the pattern called 'saddleback fever'. A week usually finds the patient convalescing, although s/he may be debilitated for the next several weeks, and some patients report unusual fatigue months later. Mortality from such classic dengue is very low.

A severe form of dengue, dengue hemorrhagic fever, occurs largely in children, and may be fatal in up to 30 percent of the cases. Sharing the symptoms of classic dengue, hemorrhagic dengue may then proceed into a state of shock, with circulatory failure, multiple hemorrhages, and sometimes death. The liver may be enlarged, and there are cases of jaundice and gastrointestinal hemorrhage, making differentiation from yellow fever difficult. This severe variant of dengue was originally found in Southeast Asia, but has now appeared in Venezuela, Columbia, India and Cuba. In Southeast Asia it is among the leading causes of hospital admission for children, and a prominent infectious cause of

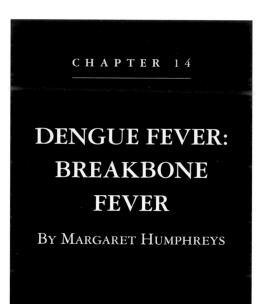

CHAPTER 14

DENGUE FEVER: BREAKBONE FEVER

By Margaret Humphreys

Cartoon of a giant mosquito swarm, spearing their victims while others flee.

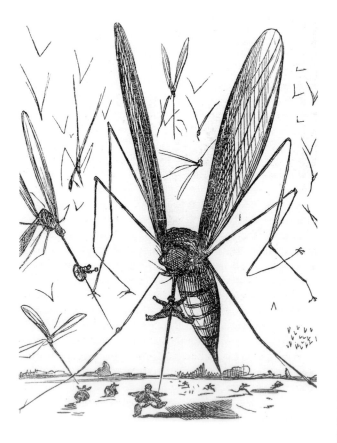

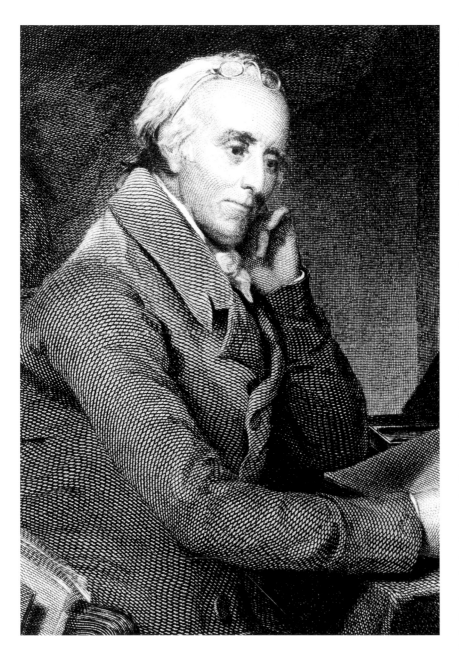

offer a person venturing into a dengue-infested area is advice about avoiding mosquito bites.

Dengue was first recognized in 1779 and 1780, on three separate continents. American physician Benjamin Rush described an outbreak in Philadelphia in the summer of 1780, which he called bilious remittent fever. He is generally credited with being the first to publish the description of dengue. The name itself comes from the Swahili *Ki denga pepo*, which refers to the sudden onset of cramps and illness caused by an evil spirit. English-speakers learned of the term from reports on the epidemic outbreak of 1827 and 1828 in the Spanish West Indies. The label 'breakbone fever' was first recorded in the 1780 Philadelphia eruption. A similar epidemic occurred in the Dutch East Indies in 1779, where David Bylon, a Dutch physician, labeled the outbreak *knokkel-koorts* (knuckle-fever). This may have been dengue, although the prominence of joint pain (knuckles included) suggests the possibility that it was another mosquito-borne disease, Chikungunya fever. There are reports of a fever in Africa from 1779 and 1780 which also resembles dengue.

Rush's description of the 1780 epidemic is, deservedly, a classic of medical observation. He begins by reporting on the climatic background, noting that 'July and August were uncommonly warm. The mercury stood on the 6th of August at $94\frac{1}{2}°$, on the 15th of the same month at $95°$, and for several days afterwards at $90°$.'

American physician Benjamin Rush (1746–1813), signer of the Declaration of Independence and prominent medical researcher, teacher and practitioner in Philadelphia during the 1790s.

death. It is now believed that the severity of dengue hemorrhagic fever is explained by the hyperactive role of the immune system; this syndrome appears most often in a patient who has been previously infected with another serotype, so that the immune response is heightened, although in ways deleterious to the patient.

Treatment for dengue is characterized by the adjective 'supportive'. There is no specific therapy that even the most modern medical center can offer the unfortunate victim of dengue. But the symptoms can be alleviated. Analgesics to control pain, aspirin or acetaminophen to bring down fever, and fluids to prevent dehydration all make the patient's course easier. In the hemorrhagic form, intravenous fluids can help with the state of shock, and support with blood products may prevent fatal hemorrhage. The only protection a physician can

Many people were ill of the heat, and a variety of diseases prevailed. Winds blowing over the docks and streets of Philadelphia filled the air with noxious odors. Most presciently Rush reported: 'The moschetoes were uncommonly numerous during the autumn.'

After setting the stage Rush goes on to give a description of dengue that matches that found in modern textbooks.

'The pains which accompanied this fever were exquisitely severe in the head, back and limbs. The pains in the head were sometimes in the back parts of it, and at other times they occupied only the eyeballs. In some people, the pains were so acute in their backs and hips, that they could not lie in bed ... A few complained of their flesh being sore to the touch, in every part of the body. From these circumstances, the disease was sometimes believed to

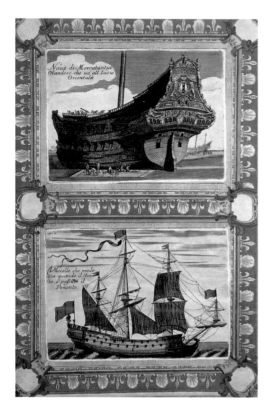

Merchant ships belonging to the Dutch East Indies Company. An epidemic in the Dutch East Indies in 1779 was labelled knuckle-fever by one physician.

be a rheumatism; but its more general name among all classes of people was the *breakbone fever.*'

Rush noted other symptoms such as nausea, rash, a quick pulse and sometimes diarrhea. He may also have seen cases of dengue hemorrhagic fever, for he recorded that in some patients, 'a profuse hæmaorrhage from the nose, mouth and bowels, on the tenth and eleventh days, preceded a fatal issue of the disease'.

Although Rush noted that the fever declined 'about the beginning of October [when] the weather became cold, accompanied by rain and an easterly wind', he failed to draw any conclusions about causation from this fact. It is now evident that lower temperatures suppress mosquito activity, but it took physicians over a hundred years to realize that this explained the tapering off of yellow fever, malaria and dengue with the onset of cold weather. Rush treated his patients with a 'gentle vomit of tartar emetic' to empty the stomach, and a purgative to cleanse the bowels, all in order to discharge the bilious matter felt to be dangerous to the patient. In addition he recommended bed rest and a liquid diet consisting of tea, lemonade, wine and apple juice. Rush allowed his patients a liberal supply of opium in order to relieve their pains. He rarely used bloodletting, the

treatment that would be so associated with his name after the 1793 yellow fever epidemic.

Rush is well known in medical history for his interest in mental disorders, and he did not fail to note the peculiar depression that followed dengue fever. After describing various other symptoms that occurred during the recovery period, he continued:

'The most remarkable symptom of the convalescence from this fever was an uncommon dejection of the spirits. I attended two young ladies, who shed tears while they vented their complaints of their sickness and weakness. One of them very aptly proposed to me to change the name of the disease, and to call it, in its present stage, instead of the breakbone, the *breakheart fever.*'

Rush tried various remedies to help such cases, but 'saw the best effects from temperate meals of oysters, and a liberal use of porter'. In line with modern medical management of fatigue and depression, he also recommended 'gentle exercise in the open air'.

Although the epidemic in Philadelphia may have been the best described, it was by no means a singular phenomenon in 1780. The fact that several outbreaks occurred nearly simultaneously makes it likely that the virus and its various vectors had been distributed worldwide through the tropics for more than 200 years. The first epidemics occurred at intervals of ten to forty years, because transmission was limited to sailing ships, and would have frequently been interrupted. Dengue probably maintained a low endemic presence in many tropical areas, made evident only by the arrival of visitors, for the natives in the place would have become immune during childhood. Epidemics would follow either when dengue was introduced to a disease-free urban

Philadelphia waterworks. The label 'breakbone fever' was first recorded in the 1780 Philadelphia outbreak.

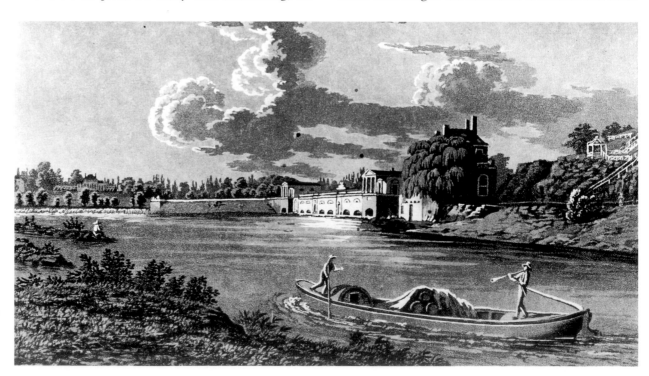

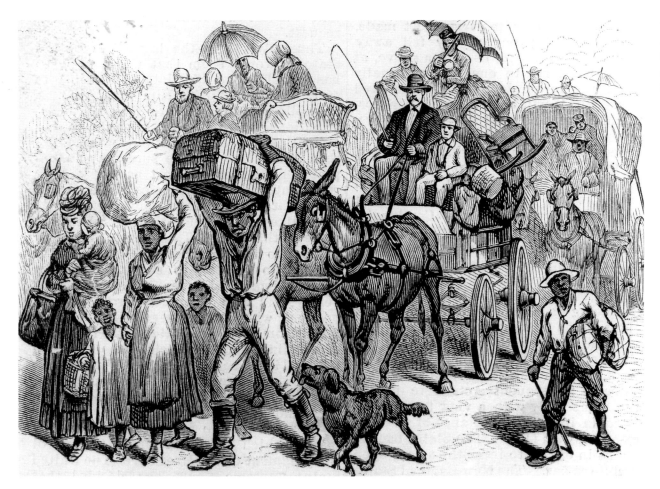

'Fleeing Mississippi'. In 1897 a puzzling outbreak of fever struck Ocean Springs, Mississippi: was it dengue fever?

area, or when a new serotype arrived in a population immune to some other form of dengue.

While classic dengue has a low mortality rate, it is similar enough to other fearsome diseases, including yellow fever, to have had a historical impact beyond its importance as a cause of death. The geographic distribution of dengue is much like that of yellow fever, which is not surprising given that they are carried by the same mosquito. Hence dengue, like yellow fever, is a disease of summer and fall in subtropical climates where the mosquito's activity is limited by the ambient temperature. So if a community was on nervous watch for yellow fever, the first cases of dengue which appeared in midsummer might cause as much panic as the real thing. There was no clear diagnostic sign for either disease in the nineteenth century, but the diagnosis of the first cases of yellow fever was critical to the implementation of quarantine. Since this would mean the isolation of a community and considerable commercial loss, local physicians were under pressure to diagnose anything but yellow fever. So, such initial cases were often frequently disputed, with competing diagnoses of dengue, hepatitis, alcoholic liver disease and malaria all vying for recognition. Physicians in nearby towns who wished to protect their communities (and perhaps increase their town's trade as well) were quick to see yellow fever elsewhere, call for quarantines, and accuse their colleagues of dishonesty.

The confusion a dengue epidemic could cause is well illustrated by events on the Gulf of Mexico coast in the 1890s. In 1897, for example, public health officials in the United States were widely criticized for letting a yellow fever epidemic on the Gulf coast go uncontrolled. By the time authorities had stepped in, the disease had spread to Louisiana, Alabama and Florida. It was a puzzling epidemic, for when it began in Ocean Springs, Mississippi there were several hundred cases before the first death occurred. Local physicians said the disease was dengue. Visiting crowds of experts for nearby state boards of health announced it was yellow fever, and that it had already spread. Altogether nine states were affected by the outbreak, with over 4,000 cases and 500 deaths. The region was terrorized, and the southern coast was blanketed with quarantine. As one physician noted at the time, the most likely cause of this unusual outbreak was a combination of yellow fever and dengue; surely the initial run of cases in Ocean Springs looked much more like dengue in its initial presentation.

Similar events happened in 1898, when American troops were clustered in camps on the Gulf and Atlantic coasts during the Spanish-American War. That summer was marked by outbreaks of typhoid, malaria and dengue. After yellow fever had been diagnosed in Mississippi and Louisiana in July, an epidemic of fever at Key West, Florida generated much excitement. There was great fear that the proximity of non-immune northern troops to the yellow fever-infested island of Cuba would lead to a major yellow fever epidemic. So when fever did occur in the Key West barracks, a nervous naval physician labeled it yellow fever, although local and federal public health officials familiar with that disease disagreed. By the time the epidemic had run its course, there had been 6,000 cases but no deaths, making dengue, not yellow fever, the likely diagnosis. The navy pulled its men out of Key West anyway, taking them to more northern bases and spreading dengue along the way.

It was not long after the mosquito vectors of yellow fever and malaria were identified in 1897 and 1900 respectively, that researchers established that dengue, too, was carried by mosquitoes. A study was published in 1906 describing experiments using human volunteers and *Aedes aegypti* mosquitoes, which demonstrated that dengue could be transmitted by mosquito bites. In 1907 two physicians proved that the causative agent was present in finely filtered blood, meaning that it was smaller than bacteria and probably belonged to the newly recognized category of viruses. An American army physician found that other *Aedes* species, including *Aedes albopictus,* could spread dengue. His work in the Philippines would have direct relevance on troop strength in the Pacific Theater during World War II. Even if dengue did not often kill soldiers, it made them ill for a week and the prolonged convalescence kept them off duty for weeks to follow.

The incidence of dengue has been increasing rapidly in the past three decades throughout the tropical regions of Asia, the Pacific, the American continents and Africa. One infectious disease specialist estimated recently that over 1.5 billion persons live in areas where dengue is a risk, and that millions of cases occur each year. Since dengue resembles many other fevers, including malaria, it is difficult to get reliable figures. Sure diagnosis can be made with serologic testing, but this precision is unavailable or unaffordable in the impoverished tropical areas most favored by dengue. Experimental trials of dengue vaccine are underway, and offer hope for the control of this debilitating, and sometimes deadly, disease.

The reasons for this resurgence are multiple. The first is the failure, worldwide, of comprehensive mosquito control. Efforts were initiated in the 1950s, based on spraying with DDT, to eradicate *Aedes aegypti* from the western hemisphere, and *Anopheles* mosquitoes (malaria carriers) from many parts of the world. As the toxic effects of DDT to the environment came to be appreciated, DDT spraying declined in popularity, although it is still in use in some tropical areas. No safe insecticide which can be used on a massive scale has been found to replace it, and mosquitoes have surged back to their pre-spraying levels everywhere. Mosquito control is underfunded in developed countries and may be non-existent in the impoverished nations where mosquito-borne diseases are most prevalent. The last few decades have seen explosive urbanization and uncontrolled population growth in developing countries, resulting in an ideal situation for dengue to spread. Substandard housing, inadequate water supplies and primitive waste management systems all support increased *Aedes* population densities. Airplanes make it easier for dengue-laden bodies and the relevant mosquitoes to be rapidly transported from one locale to another. This, coupled

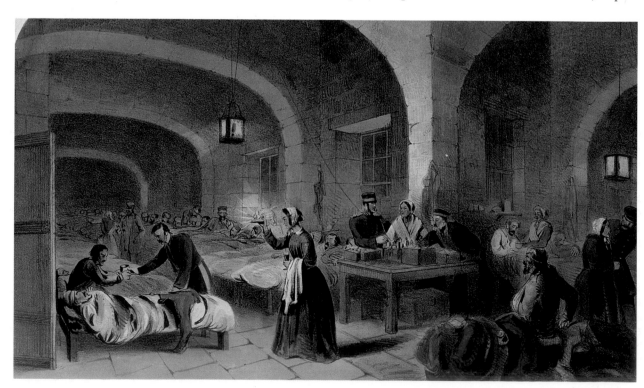

Florence Nightingale at her field hospital at Scutari: battlefield fevers were notoriously difficult to diagnose.

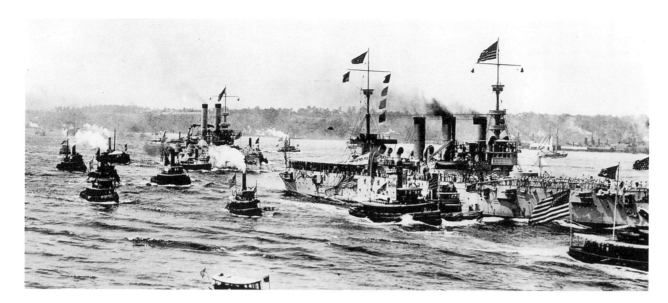

Spanish American War. US fleet returning to the States in 1898. USS New York is followed in column by USS Iowa.

with inadequate surveillance, can lead to the virus establishing a beachhead before its presence has even been noticed.

Although hemorrhagic dengue can be an important cause of death, in its classic form dengue is identified as a 'benign' disease because most of its victims survive. But it is far from benign in its economic and social impact. The concern over hemorrhagic dengue led to the hospitalization of over 700,000 children in Southeast Asia in the past thirty years, making it an important cause of rising health costs. In Thailand it is estimated that in 1980 dengue alone cost nearly seven million dollars in hospitalization and mosquito control. Similar costs were incurred in American epidemics. During 1977, when Puerto Rico was overwhelmed by a dengue epidemic, over ten million dollars was devoured by medical costs, control measures, loss of productive labor and damage to the tourist industry. In the ten years that followed dengue returned eight times, multiplying this loss to over a hundred million dollars. Cuba was similarly afflicted in 1981, but reported that with the expenditure of over a hundred million dollars the epidemic was stopped, and *Aedes aegypti* rates reduced to vanishing numbers. There is no reason to think that dengue will be any less of a problem in the future.

BIBLIOGRAPHY

Gubler, Duane. J. 1988. 'Dengue', in Thomas P. Monath (ed.), *The Arboviruses: Epidemiology and Ecology*, vol. II, pp. 223–54. Boca Raton, Florida.

Gubler, Duane J. and Gary G. Clark. 1995. 'Dengue/Dengue Hemorrhagic Fever: The Emergence of a Global Health Problem', *Journal of Emerging Diseases*, vol. 2 (via the internet).

Halstead, Scott B. 1994. 'Dengue', in Paul D. Hoeprich et al.(eds.), *Infectious Diseases* (5th edn), pp. 919–23.

Humphreys, Margaret. 1992. Yellow Fever and the South. New Brunswick, New Jersey; 1995. 'Imported Dengue-United States, 1993–1994', *Morbidity and Mortality Weekly Report*, vol. 44, pp. 35–36.

McSherry, James. 1993. 'Dengue', in Kenneth F. Kiple (ed.), *The Cambridge World History of Human Disease*. Cambridge, England and New York.

Rush, Benjamin. 1815 (1st pub. 1789). 'An Account of the Bilious Remitting Fever, as it appeared in Philadelphia in the Summer and Autumn of the year 1780', in *Medical Inquiries and Observations* (4th edn), vol. II, pp. 231–9. Philadelphia.

The army's DDT bomb is now used in the home. Mrs Goldstein of Brooklyn, New York, using the spray to kill insects. Her son watches, illustrating the safety of the spray.

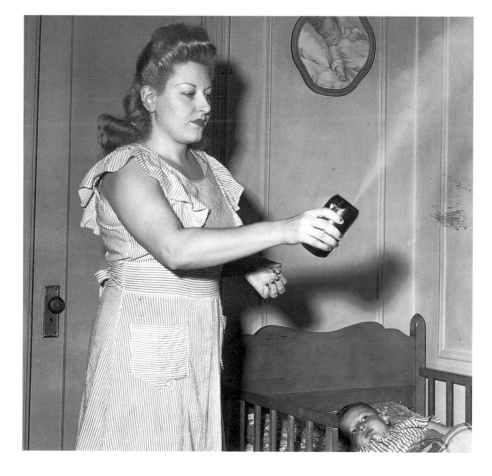

CHAPTER 15

MALARIA: 'EVIL' AIR AND MOSQUITOES

BY MARGARET HUMPHREYS

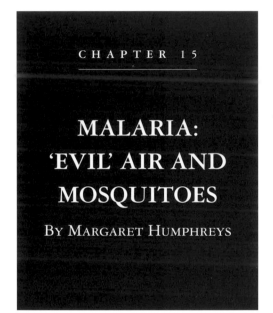

Malaria is one of the greatest plagues of humankind. Even though it does not kill often, it robs people of their energy, their capacity to enjoy life, their ability to make a living. Malaria is caused by microorganisms called plasmodia, and many kinds of animals have a particular species of plasmodium all of their own. It may be that the malaria parasite got its start as a single-celled plant like the algae, for the organism's DNA shows evidence that an ancestor could manufacture chlorophyll, the substance that makes plants green and allows for photosynthesis. Four species of plasmodia infect humans, and cause untold misery: *vivax*, *falciparum*, *malariae* and *ovale*, with the first two generating the majority of cases. *Falciparum* is the most severe, and may cause death. The other three types of malaria are relatively mild, although they generate very uncomfortable symptoms and may lead to chronic anemia and weakness.

Malaria leaves no marks on bones, which means that there is nothing for archaeologists to find in skeletal remains that would prove malaria's antiquity. However, we can draw some conclusions about the ancient origin and distribution of the disease from contemporary evidence. For example, it is likely that the malaria parasite moved from monkeys to humans. Since the highest density of simian malarias is in South Asia (and rare among African monkeys) that may be a sign that the disease first moved into humans in Thailand or India. Another indicator is the presence of genetic traits for the resistance of malaria, which serve as evidence that the disease has prevailed in that population over enough generations for the traits to be amplified by natural selection. Given that New World native peoples show no adaptations to resist malaria, it is at least possible that human malaria first appeared in South Asia, migrated to Africa and Europe, and thence to the Americas. It is unlikely that malaria survived the trek across the Russia–Alaska land bridge, because there are no records of the illness in any of the ancient Indian writings, and no signs of biological adaptation among Native American peoples.

Such signs are present in peoples from Africa, the Mediterranean countries and India. The malaria parasite attacks the red blood cells, and modifications in the structure of those cells seem to protect against infection. Sickle cell is the most well-known of these blood cell anomalies. It represents an interesting bargain with the forces of life and death. Babies born with genes for sickle cell from both parents will die at an early age unless modern medical intervention is available. Babies with no sickle cell genes at all are at risk of dying young from malaria. But those lucky tots with only one gene have both protection against malaria, and almost no symptoms from their aberrant blood-cell trait. Other changes in peoples from these regions also protect against malaria, so effectively that many of those of African descent cannot be infected with *vivax* malaria at all.

Malaria was known as intermittent or remittent fever in the past, because of its peculiar cycle of symptoms. The patient first notices a freezing chill, as if immersed in ice water. As the fever soars to 104 or even 106°, awareness of great heat follows. Then the patient collapses with exhaustion, sweating rivers while the temperature drops back to normal. In simple *vivax* malaria, this cycle will then be repeated like clockwork, every forty-eight hours. This pattern of day one, day three led to the name 'tertian fever'. *Vivax* was benign tertian fever; *falciparum* was malignant tertian fever. Since *vivax* (for reasons still not clear) tends to appear in the spring, and *falciparum* in the summer and fall, the former might be called 'vernal fever', and the latter 'aestivoautumnal fever'. Repeated bouts of malaria caused extensive red blood cell destruction, and hence anemia.

Malaria is carried by *anopheles* mosquitoes. It is the female mosquito who bites, seeking a blood meal to develop her eggs; the male spends his time sipping nectar and looking for sex. After being sucked up from a malaria patient by the mosquito, the parasite goes through part of its life-cycle in the insect's gut, and then makes its way to the mosquito's salivary glands, ready to be injected when she takes her next meal. After entering into a new human host, the parasite travels first to the liver, multiplies enormously, attacks red

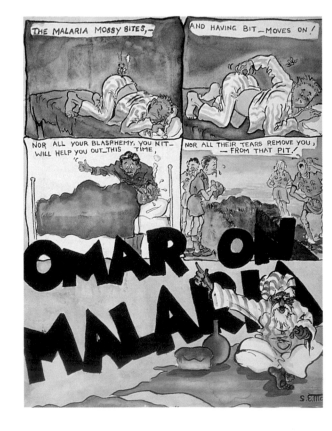

Satirical sketches about malaria. Coloured pen drawings by S. E. Moyer, 1943.

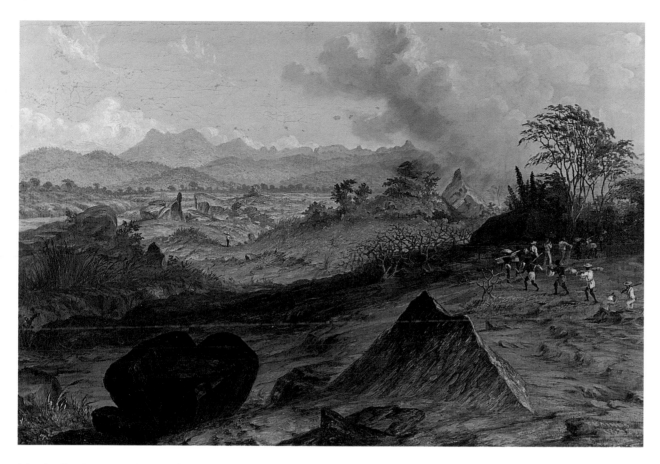

blood cells, changes and multiplies again, and then emerges ready to be picked up by the next feeding mosquito.

Malaria has been a major disease in sub-Saharan Africa, the Near East and the Asian tropics throughout recorded history; it also flourished in Europe and China well into modern times. In China it was known as 'Mother of Fevers', and the author of the 2700 BC medical classic *Nei Ching* described the cyclic fevers and enlarged spleen of malaria accurately. The cuneiform writings of the Sumerians and Vedic writings of 1600 BC similarly make it clear that malaria was a significant health problem in the ancient world. Some have even traced the demise of the Greek and Roman civilizations to the enervating effects of the malaria parasite.

Ancient writers were quick to notice the correlation of swamps and malaria. Some, like Hippocrates, said drinking such stagnant water caused malaria; others worried that the foul air emanating from swamps poisoned the system and caused fever. The disease was known under many names, including 'swamp fever', 'ague' and 'Roman fever', because the marshy lands around Rome seemed so productive of the sickness. The name 'malaria' itself came from the Italian, meaning 'evil air'. The first specific use of the term may have been by Horace Walpole, who in a letter home from Italy in 1740 described 'A horrid thing called mal'aria that comes to Rome every summer and kills one.' Until the late nineteenth century 'malaria' was used to mean the cause of the disease, not the disease itself.

During the age of exploration malaria was widespread in Europe as well as Africa. While *falciparum* is limited to the tropics, *vivax* is more tolerant of cold, and has appeared as far north as England and southern Canada. So it is likely that many *vivax* parasites traveled in European bodies to the New World, while *falciparum* came inside Africans making the horrid Middle Passage. While *vivax* was a nuisance that limited the capacity to work, *falciparum* raged within Europeans who tried to live in the tropics, leaving them shivering, burning and sometimes dying from this fierce 'new' ague. *Falciparum* malaria helped dig the 'White Man's Grave' of the West African coast; only the relative inefficiency of the American mosquito vector kept the Caribbean from being equally deadly to Europeans. But the difference was only relative – *falciparum* made mortality high enough to threaten even the bravest colonizer. Their African slaves, on the other hand, had inborn genetic traits that helped them survive *falciparum*'s ravages and, ironically, made them all the more efficient as carriers. It was just this resistance to malaria that made African slaves even more valuable, since white indentured labor could not survive and produce under the Caribbean sun.

Paradoxically the New World offered one of the first effective drugs for malaria, even though the disease made its appearance there relatively late in history. Jesuit missionaries returning home to Spain from Peru brought with them a powdered bark that was remarkably good for fevers. Scientists in the nineteenth century extracted the potent compound in the bark of the *cinchona* tree, and named it quinine. It became the mainstay of malaria therapy in the west until new drugs were developed in the twentieth century. China had its own native malaria remedy called 'Qinghuasu', which is derived from the sweet wormwood plant, *Artemisia annua*. As parasites have become increasingly resistant to western medicines in recent years, pharmaceutical industry interest in Qinghuasu (extracted and purified as artemisinin) has grown, resulting in recent field trials in Thailand, where it was effective in treating patients with drug-resistant malaria.

By the nineteenth century the idea that malaria was caused by inhaling swampy air or drinking swamp water was firmly entrenched. This allowed communities to take measures to control the disease, even though their etiological theory was faulty. Drainage of standing water did help – not by vaporizing the foul air, of course, but by destroying mosquito breeding areas. The town of Savannah, for example, managed in the early nineteenth century to cut its malaria rate significantly by ruling that rice fields could not be sown near the town. They also planted trees to serve as a screen against the miasmata, or foul airs, that blew in from the fields and swampy areas. All probably had the effect of reducing *anopheles* density, so city officials were pleased at the good results, and believed the miasm theory about poisonous air vindicated. Many other cities also pursued drainage programs, with the combined intentions of liberating land for development, and suppressing the malarious miasms.

In the last two decades of the nineteenth century a revolution occurred in the understanding of infectious diseases. Robert Koch, Louis Pasteur and their followers convinced the world that infections were caused by microorganisms. The germs of tuberculosis, anthrax, cholera, diphtheria, typhoid and so on, were found, one after another. Two investigators working in Italy even claimed to have found the malaria bacillus, living appropriately enough in the swamp mud of a highly malarious area. This bacterium gained acceptance for a while, but by 1886 a new contender for the cause of malaria was gaining recognition.

It was found by an unlikely hero, a French army surgeon stationed in Algeria, who looked at slide after slide of malarious blood under the microscope. Alphonse Laveran repeatedly saw an odd ring of black pigment in the red blood cells, and often also crescent-shaped black bodies. In a bold move he announced that this (or these) were the malaria parasites. But how could so many different shaped things be one microorganism? It took a leap of imagination to recognize that the parasite went through stages of its life cycle in the human body, assuming different shapes at different times in its life. Leading figures of the time were slow to accept Laveran's germ – Robert Koch scoffed at it, as did William Osler, the dean of American medicine. Laveran was hampered by his inability to explain how the parasite moved from one body to another. He searched the soil and water of malarious Algeria hoping to find the answer, but failed.

Some factor had to explain the proximity of malaria to swamps, and if the organism was not in the water, where was it? Several physicians began to suspect that it might be in mosquitoes. Patrick Manson of the London School of

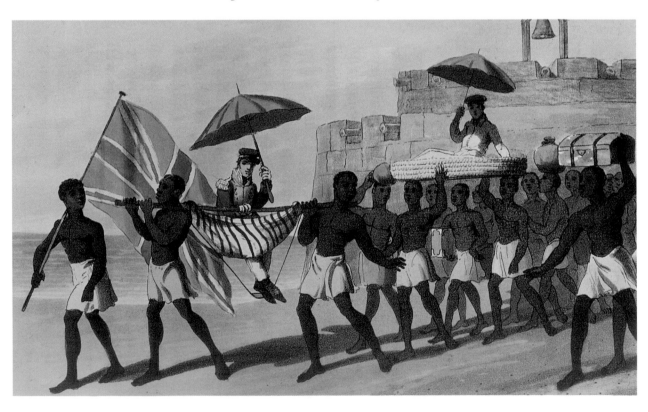

Traveling in Africa – W. Hutton, Voyage to Africa, 1821, Royal Geographic Society.

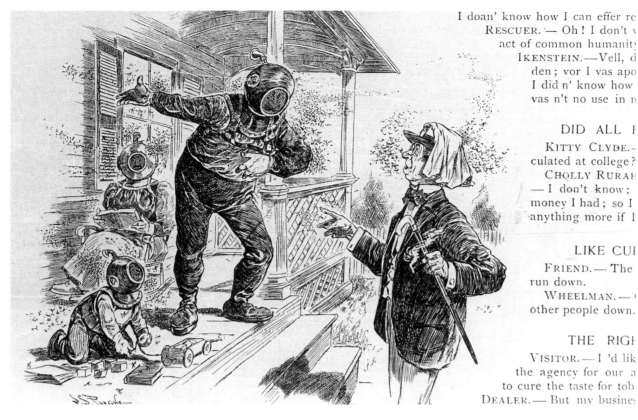

I doan' know how I can effer re
RESCUER. — Oh! I don't v
act of common humanit;
IKENSTEIN. — Vell, d
den; vor I vas apo
I did n' know how
vas n't no use in n

DID ALL I
KITTY CLYDE.-
culated at college?
CHOLLY RURAF
— I don't know;
money I had; so I
anything more if I

LIKE CUI
FRIEND. — The
run down.
WHEELMAN. —
other people down.

THE RIGI
VISITOR. — I 'd lik
the agency for our a
to cure the taste for tob
DEALER. — But my busine;

'Sundown in the Suburbs'. A cartoon showing life in an American suburb plays on the idea of air-borne diseases.

Tropical Medicine and Hygiene had established that filariasis, a tropical worm disease, was spread by mosquitoes. Manson suspected malaria might be as well, and he supported British army physician Ronald Ross, stationed in India, in his attempt to establish such transmission. As every British schoolchild knows, Ross did so in 1897. He proved that avian malaria was transmitted from bird to bird by mosquitoes. While Ross wanted to go on to work on human malaria, he was prevented by the army's bureaucracy, which transferred him away from the malarious region where his work had begun.

But Ross had done enough to set off a revolution in the understanding of malaria and its control, and he won the Nobel Prize for his demonstration in 1907. A year after Ross's avian work, Italian scientists established that human malaria was transmitted in the same way. This concept was put to practical use a few years later, when it was shown that workers on the Panama Canal could be kept nearly free of malaria by controlling the mosquito population, treating cases with quinine, and protecting human bodies from mosquitoes by means of nets and screens.

Much information about malaria emerged from this initial research. More was to come from an unlikely source – attempts at treating the late stages of syphilis. Tertiary syphilis causes severe disease of the nervous system, resulting in muscle weakness, insanity and death. Although by the 1910s there was a drug available to treat syphilis, Paul Ehrlich's famous salvarsan, it was not very useful for the late stages. Julius Wagner von Juarreg, a Viennese

psychiatrist, noted that the syphilis treponeme was very susceptible to heat, and wondered whether giving neurosyphilis patients a fever would improve their condition. After trying tuberculin and other substances, he found that injection of live *vivax* parasites produced the most satisfactory results. He let the patients go through several cycles of high fever, and then treated the malaria with quinine. For this work he won the Nobel Prize in 1927, and the technique was used widely until penicillin became available after World War II. It was from this therapy that physicians were able to establish differential susceptibility to malaria infection. In a mental hospital in the Florida panhandle repeated attempts were made to infect black patients with *vivax*, but finally it had to be admitted that only *falciparum* would 'take', and that only produced really satisfactory fevers if the patient did not have prior infection.

However the principal focus of malaria researchers was on methods of prevention, which caused much controversy. Robert Koch believed that malaria could be controlled with quinine alone, if given in sufficient quantity and for long enough. Ross himself thought that rigorous mosquito control, through the destruction or alteration of breeding areas, would be sufficient. This debate over combating the mosquito versus attacking the plasmodium directly has dominated twentieth-century discourse about malaria control. A key element is the relative cost of the two types of measures, for the countries most troubled by malaria are often those that have the least to spend on health improvement schemes.

Both avenues of action were tried with varying success in several places around the world. By the end of the 1930s it was widely acknowledged among malariologists that no single method worked well everywhere, and in some areas, such as Africa, nothing made very significant inroads into the malaria problem. But in the 1940s all this changed. A new weapon was at hand: DDT. This compound had been synthesized in 1877, but only in the 1940s did entomologists come to realize what a potent insecticide it was. DDT had an amazing property. Not only did spraying it on walls kill a wide variety of insects, including mosquitoes, but it continued to destroy insects who landed on a sprayed surface for up to three months. Since anopheline mosquitoes almost always land on walls to rest after taking a blood meal, if houses were sprayed with DDT the malaria chain could be effectively broken. And after World War II DDT was cheap and widely available. Millions of dwellings all over the world were sprayed, and malaria declined at rates never seen before.

This optimistic picture led the World Health Organization to declare in 1955, that with DDT and the world's support, they could eradicate malaria from the globe. Broad swathes of India and other tropical countries became malaria-free, and hope surged that the demise of humankind's ancient enemy was near. But then troubling news started coming in from the field.

Mosquitoes were developing resistance to DDT. And by the early 1960s, when Rachel Carson published her clarion call for the environmental movement, *Silent Spring*, it became no longer possible to ignore the toxicity of DDT and other pesticides. DDT spraying began to decline, and malaria made its comeback.

There was initial hope that this resurgence might be controlled with effective medications, and ultimately a vaccine. After World War II chloroquine was introduced, and remains a mainstay of malaria prevention and treatment. It is much better tolerated than quinine, and more therapeutically active against the malaria parasite. It also works to prevent acquisition of the disease, if the parasite is sensitive to it. Other drugs were developed in the 1950s and 1960s that were equally successful. But again, bad news arrived to disrupt the optimism that had been created. In the first place, impoverished peoples could not afford the drugs. Beyond that limitation, which might have been overcome by international funding, emerged a worse problem. The organism was becoming resistant, and at a rapid rate. Nowadays there are malaria parasites that are impervious to all modern drugs, although they still respond somewhat to quinine. Attempts at making a vaccine met with failure. Only recently has a vaccine that works at all been developed, and even that one, generated by the best of modern medical research, is not predictably effective.

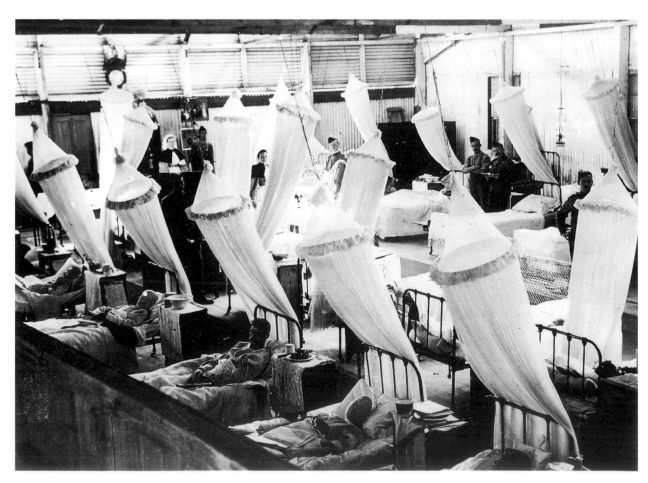

A ward in a South African hospital during the Boer War. Note the mosquito netting over the beds.

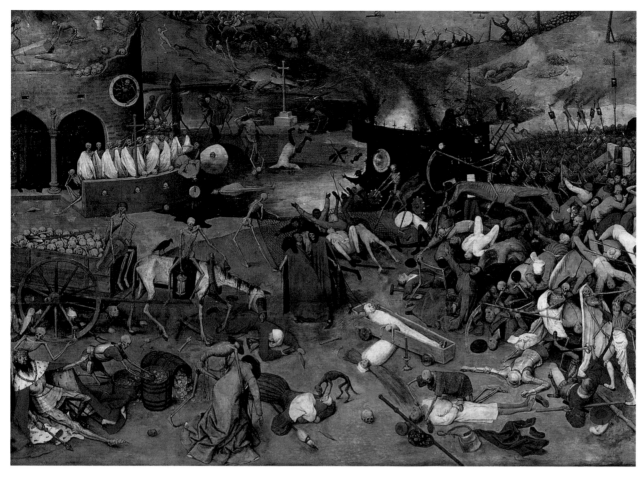

In 'The Triumph of Death', c. 1562, by Pieter the Elder Breughel (1515–69), the 'fumes' ultimately overcome all.

Poster warning against malaria mosquitoes and urging protection from their bites.

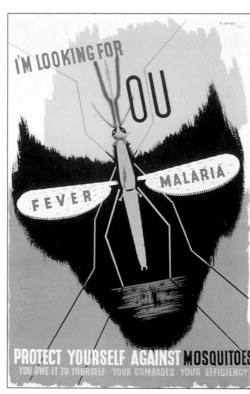

In 1969 the World Health Organization had to admit that the plan to eradicate malaria had failed, and that a more realistic goal was to attempt improvement in the worst areas. While the disease has not returned to its haunts in Europe, the United States or Canada, it has flourished anew in the American, African and Asian tropics, where it causes more than two million deaths annually. As one malariologist summarized gloomily in 1991:

'The outlook for malaria control is grim. The disease, caused by mosquito-borne parasites, is present in 102 countries and is responsible for over a hundred million clinical cases and one to two million deaths each year. Over the past two decades, efforts to control malaria have met with less and less success. In many regions where malaria transmission had been almost eliminated, the disease has made a comeback, sometimes surpassing earlier recorded levels. The dream of completely eliminating malaria from many parts of the world, pursued with vigor during the 1950s and 1960s, has gradually faded. Few believe today that a global eradication of malaria will be possible in the - foreseeable future.'

BIBLIOGRAPHY

Ackerknecht, Erwin H. 1945. *Malaria in the Upper Mississippi Valley*, 1760–1900. Baltimore.

Bruce-Chwatt, Leonard Jan and Julian de Zulueta. 1980. *The Rise and Fall of Malaria in Europe: A Historicoepidemiological Study.* Oxford.

Desowitz, Robert S. 1991. *The Malaria Capers. More Tales of Parasites and People, Research and Reality.* New York and London.

Dunn, Frederick L. 1993. 'Malaria', in Kenneth F. Kiple (ed.), *The Cambridge World History of Human Disease.* Cambridge, England and New York.

Harrison, Gordon. 1978. *Mosquitoes, Malaria & Man: A History of the Hostilities since 1880.* New York.

Humphreys, Margaret. 1996. 'Kicking a Dying Dog: DDT and the Demise of Malaria in the American South, 1942–1952', *Isis 87*, pp. 1–17.

Oaks, Stanley C. et al. (eds.). 1991. *Malaria: Obstacles and Opportunities.* Washington, DC.

Stoute, José A. et al. 1997. 'A Preliminary Evaluation of a Recombinant Circumsporozoite Protein Vaccine against Plasmodium Falciparum Malaria', *New England Journal of Medicine*, vol. 336, pp. 86–91.

In the past, typhus was known by names like 'ship's fever', 'camp fever', 'war fever' and 'jail fever'. Clearly the infection was associated with crowded and unhygienic conditions. Through a wider lens, however, typhus was viewed as a disease of disasters. The German epidemiologist August Hirsch, writing in the nineteenth century, lamented that 'the history of typhus ... is the history of human misery'. He connected the malady with famines as well as wars and revolutions that brought about times of want, especially when those events occurred in cold weather. But although much was known for hundreds of years about the circumstances likely to summon typhus, knowledge of its cause came only in the twentieth century.

CHAPTER 16

TYPHUS, SHIPS AND SOLDIERS

By Kenneth F. Kiple and Kriemhild Coneè Ornelas

In 1934 Hans Zinsser, a bacteriologist who studied typhus in the century's earlier decades, introduced many readers to the history of the malady in his rambling, but delightful scrutiny of *Rats, Lice, and History*. The book's title identifies two of the culprits indirectly responsible for infecting humans with the illness. Those directly responsible, the pathogens, whose transmission rats and lice facilitate, are neither viruses nor bacteria but rather *Rickettsia* – microorganisms midway between the two. One species of the pathogen is transmitted by the rat flea and causes murine (or endemic) typhus; another mite-borne type carries scrub typhus (Tsutsugamushi disease); and still another related illness is Rocky Mountain Spotted Fever, passed along through ticks. But the reputation as the most widespread and deadly of the rickettsial organisms belongs to epidemic typhus. This form of the disease has killed millions of people and, by deciding battles and overturning rulers and their empires, has changed the course of history many times over the centuries.

Epidemic typhus is caused by the microorganism *Rickettsia prowazekii*, which is passed along from person to person by the human body louse (*Pediculus humanus corporis*) and sometimes by the human head louse (*Pediculus humanus capitis*).

Body lice depend on humans to shelter them and their eggs in their clothing, warm them with their bodies, and feed them with their blood – all reasons why heaven for the little creatures historically has consisted of soldiers, or sailors, crowded together in cold weather, wearing a considerable amount of clothing but with little opportunity for changing it. Such conditions are also ideal for the spread of typhus pathogens. They are ingested by the lice with blood meals from infected persons, then transmitted to other victims when the lice desert feverish or dead human hosts for individuals with more satisfactory body temperatures. Unfortunately for the lice, they get no reward for their vectorial activity. Instead,

Typhus victims kept in isolation during World War I, in Estonia.

lice infected with typhus always die, whereas most of the humans they infect (60 to 90 percent) manage to survive.

In addition to high fever, the most characteristic symptom of typhus is a widespread rash lasting for one to two weeks, as its names in German, *Fleckfieber* ('spotted fever'), and in Spanish, *tabardillo* ('red cloak'), suggest. The word typhus comes from the Greek *typhos* and was employed during ancient times to signify stupor arising from fever – a situation frequently characteristic of typhus. But it only came to mean the malady under discussion in the eighteenth century, and it was not until the middle of the nineteenth that typhus was disentangled from typhoid – a disease with similar symptoms.

All of this leads us straight into a semantical jungle that flourishes to this day. Although typhus and typhoid were separated clinically as different disease entities, their distinction did not necessarily extend to the nosological, and, in fact, in some European languages typhus continues to mean typhoid. This confusion has, in turn, been compounded by those vague appellations already mentioned – 'jail fever', 'ship's fever' and the like which could have been typhus but could also have been any number of other infections.

Because epidemic typhus occurs as a natural infection only in humans and needs no other reservoir, a lengthy relationship is implied between the pathogen (which probably evolved from that of endemic typhus) and people. Nonetheless, the written history of the disease can only be said with assurance to have begun with the dawning of the Age of Discovery, although Hirsch and Zinsser have pointed out that an outbreak in a Salerno monastery in 1083 may well have been typhus, and some have claimed that it was this malady at

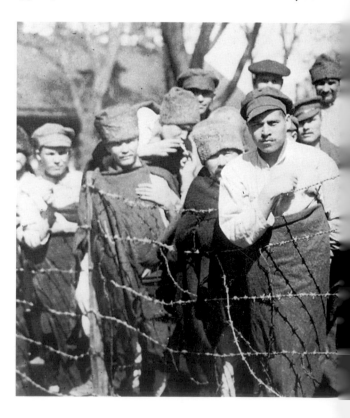

work on a Greek battlefield in 430 BC which went down in history as the mysterious 'Plague of Athens'.

But despite the possibility of earlier debuts in European history, there is considerable agreement that the years 1489–90 mark the time that typhus arrived in Europe to take up permanent residence. It appeared during the last spasms of an eight-hundred-year struggle by the Iberians to reconquer their peninsula from the Moors, when Spanish soldiers at Gianada suddenly found themselves under assault by more than Moors. The disease so abruptly in their midst killed 17,000 of them – six times more than their human enemies had managed.

The infection in question had definite typhus-like symptoms (a Spanish chronicler called the disease 'a malignant spotted fever'); it apparently arrived with troops from Cyprus, 'an island in which this fever was prevalent'; and it revealed a typhus-like affinity for battlefields. In short, it seems to have been the same disease that would frequent so many of them over the next few centuries.

Typhus moved swiftly in establishing itself and within the next decade had become ensconced in Italy, where in 1528 it made another battlefield appearance – this time with history-making decisiveness and this time in the service of Spain, or at least the King of Spain, Carlos I, who was also Charles V of the Holy Roman Empire.

A little earlier, under Ferdinand and Isabella, Spain had fought with France over various of the Italian principalities, and a new disease – syphilis – that broke out in late 1494 among the troops of France near Naples had forced a French withdrawal. Now, however, in 1528, the French seemed on

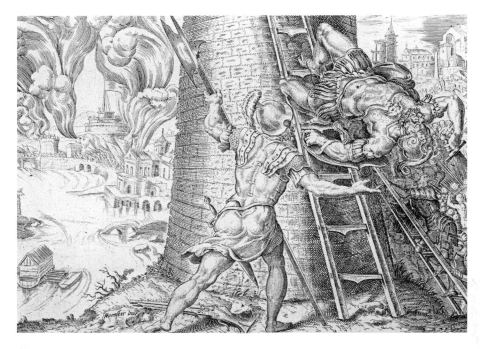

the verge of a great victory. The remnants of the Imperial forces, already ravaged by bubonic plague, and under siege near Naples, were unpaid and unhappy – barely subsisting on bread and water. The Pope and all of Italy had already written off Emperor Charles and stood ready to acknowledge the rule of Francis I of France. But, once again, Neapolitan pathogens played a pivotal role in human affairs. In July typhus counterattacked and within a month it had struck down some 30,000 soldiers, bringing about the second disastrous French retreat from Naples in four decades.

Meanwhile, typhus had also been sporadically busy outside of southern Europe. In sixteenth-century England, beginning at Cambridge in 1522, and later at Oxford and Exeter, typhus became the scourge behind the famous 'Black Assizes', during which 'jail fever', simmering amid prisoners, suddenly spread explosively among courtroom spectators, jurors and judges. In addition, before mid-century the disease had found its way into France and Germany and probably Eastern Europe.

In 1546 Girolamo Fracastoro (Fracastorius), called by some the 'father of epidemiology', published his *De Contagione...*, a chapter of which gained him credit for penning the first clear description of typhus. Yet, in the second half of the sixteenth century, it is doubtful that anyone needed a handbook on contagious diseases to

The army of Charles V at Naples, where typhus killed 30,000 soldiers on the battlefield, resulting in a surprise victory for the Spanish.

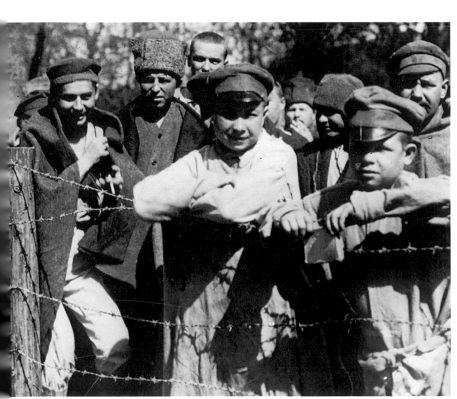

'Jack Frost attacking Bony in Russia', by William Elmes, 1812: but disease did as much to defeat Napoleon's armies as the weather.

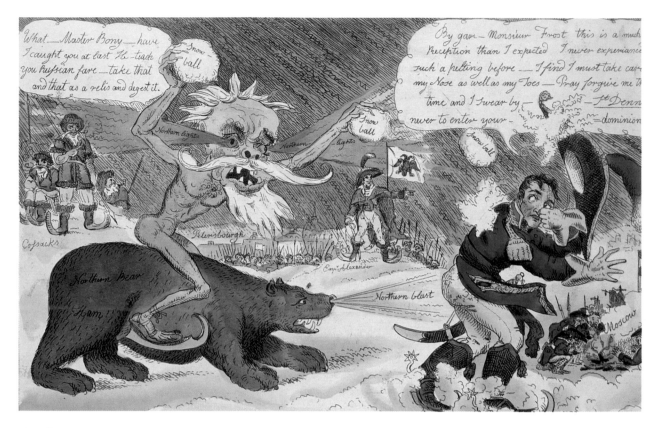

identify typhus, which suddenly had become all too familiar. In 1552 the infection joined forces with other illnesses to turn on Charles V for a change, forcing him to abandon the siege of Metz after killing 10,000 or so of his men. Soldiers, returning to their homes after the siege had been lifted, touched off typhus everywhere they went.

In the Balkans, Imperial soldiers who gathered to battle the Turks were frequently struck down by typhus before ever encountering a Turk. Some 30,000 died in 1542 alone, and Hungary became known as the 'Graveyard of Germans'. In 1566 another severe epidemic erupted to scatter some 80,000 Imperial troops of Maximilian II who were poised to attack the Sultan of Hungary. This earned typhus still another sobriquet – *morbus hungaricus* – which, along with famine, spread to engulf Austria, Germany, the Netherlands, Switzerland and, once again, Italy.

Whether typhus was present in the New World before 1492, reached it during the first days of exploration and conquest, or waited for decades before making an appearance has been the subject of debate, with some scholars convinced that this was the disease called *modorra* (drowsiness or stupor) that afflicted Spaniards at the time of the voyages of discovery of the Indies. But there is no question that, during the second half of the sixteenth century, typhus hurdled the Atlantic to join other plagues in decimating Amerindians. The disease took root in the mountainous regions of South and Central America and is alleged to have been *cocoliztli* — the plague that devastated the Mexican highlands by precipitating a death toll customarily put at two million. The Spanish

conquistadors, who were certainly no strangers to typhus, as it was by this time widespread in Iberia, and who were themselves lice-ridden – they were described as 'proud but lousy' – readily identified the massive 1576 epidemic as typhus or *tabardillo*; indeed, the very fact that the Spaniards did not get the disease while Indians were dying all around them may well indicate the immunity to the infection that can be acquired, at least for a time, by suffering through it and surviving.

In seventeenth-century Europe typhus accompanied marching armies with increasing virulence, and during the Thirty Years War (1618–48) battle casualties were minor in comparison with the damage inflicted by this malady and by other diseases such as plague, scurvy and dysentery. Civilians, too, sustained heavy losses; Germany was said to be so devastated that in some villages wolves wandered through empty streets. The Baltic Wars extended the range of typhus to the Scandinavian countries; the struggle between Crown troops and Huguenots spread it throughout France; and the infection became a major participant in the English Civil Wars. In 1643 it impartially ravaged both the Parliamentary and the Royal armies at the siege of Reading, and another epidemic in 1650 reportedly turned the entire island into one huge hospital.

In discussing the eighteenth century Hirsch wrote: 'We find scarcely a year without references to epidemics of typhus, great or small, in one part of Europe or another.' At the risk of redundancy, we might add that the 'great' epidemics were mostly associated with war. The wars of the Spanish, Polish and Austrian successions that shook the continent during the first half of the century provided fertile ground for typhus. But the wars of its second half – the Seven Years War, the French Revolution and the Napoleonic campaigns – saw the disease assume a savagery that, in comparison, made guns and bayonets seem insignificant hazards to human life.

The continental wars sheltered England from a typhus-ridden Europe, but, at the end of the century, the infection found its way southward from an Ireland plagued with famine to fuel an epidemic that, between 1816 and 1819, reached white-hot intensity in both islands. In Ireland some 700,000 persons out of a population of six million were said to have contracted the disease.

It was in 1812, however, that typhus once again appears to have changed the course of history – and once again on a battlefield. Napoleon's close to half a million soldiers marched into Russia to collide with typhus as well as the Russians. The French bad luck against the disease held, and, after the battle of Ostrowo, typhus had taken such a heavy toll as to force a retreat from Moscow. When this got underway in October 1812, only 80,000 men (less than 20 percent of those who had entered Russia) were fit for duty. Only 6,000 made it back and Napoleon's career of conquest was at an end.

Sailors as well as soldiers suffered from typhus; indeed, after scurvy, 'ships fever' was their biggest scourge. But typhus was also a 'ships fever' because ships efficiently shuttled the infection from one spot on the globe to another. The famous British naval surgeon James Lind (1716–94), considered the founder of the study of naval hygiene but better known today for his efforts to conquer scurvy, was also in the forefront of the war against 'ships fever'. His recommendations that sailors be stripped, scrubbed, shaved and issued clean clothes were acted upon, and British seamen attained a freedom from the infection not achieved by others, including their French rivals whose vessels were especially

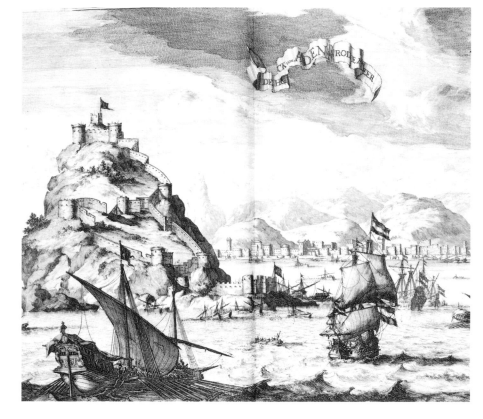

filthy and typhus-ridden. These preventive measures gave England a sizable edge in naval warfare.

As already noted, ships carried typhus to Spanish America in the sixteenth century, but the question of when it attained a presence north of Mexico remains a murky one. It is likely that the infectious fevers described by William Bradford (1590–1657), longtime governor of Plymouth Colony and author of *Plymouth Plantation*, were typhus. The fevers arrived by ship in 1629 and 1634, already well established in the midst of the passengers. The first swept Salem plantation but spared Plymouth, whereas Bradford credited the second with killing many Indians living nearby.

Following this, there are numerous reports of illnesses that could have been typhus reaching North America by ship and, as the pace of immigration quickened, so did the pace of infection. Typhus reached Philadelphia with German immigrants in 1754, precipitating an outbreak so severe that a systematic screening of arriving ships and passengers was undertaken. According to Hirsch, in the nineteenth century Irish immigrants in particular were implicated in the introduction of typhus to Canada, beginning at Halifax, Nova Scotia in 1827. Quebec

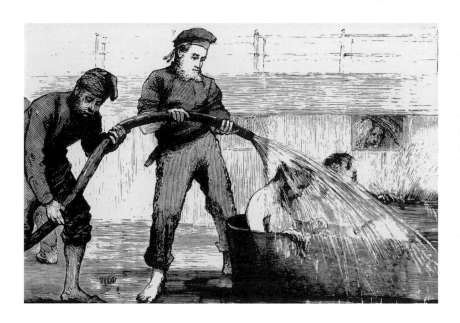

Typhus was known as 'shipboard fever' and struck in all the major port cities (like Aden, on the Arabian Sea, above). As a result of recommendations of James Lind, British sailors were stripped, scrubbed and shaved, to keep typhus at bay (left).

Japanese nurses tending the sick in the Russo–Japanese War, 1904–5.

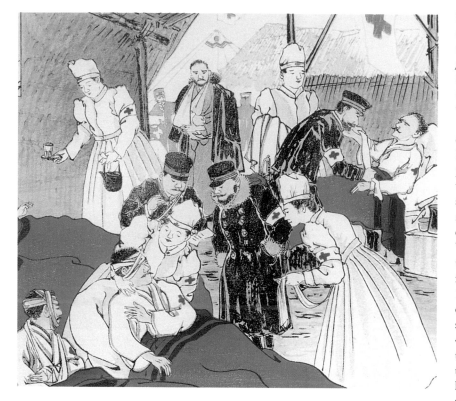

but in 1916 a Brazilian scientist confirmed Ricketts' observations and named the organism *Rickettsia prowazekii* – the species in honor of Stanislas J. M. von Prowazek, a Polish scientist, who had also died of typhus while investigating it.

During World War I, both sides employed the knowledge disclosed by Nicolle to implement delousing procedures, but a continuation of very primitive conditions in the east seemed to attract the disease like a magnet. There was not a single outbreak of epidemic typhus on the Western Front, but a holocaust of the malady in the east. In Serbia, the first six months of the war brought 150,000 typhus deaths, and other countries on the Eastern Front were similarly affected. Of the fewer than 400 doctors in Serbia, 126 died from the disease, along with fully half of the 60,000 Austrian prisoners of war held there. Yet typhus was also something of a blessing in disguise for the Serbs because, so long as the epidemic reigned, the Austrians dared not attack.

During (and especially after) the war, however, it was the Russians who suffered, almost unbelievably horribly, from typhus. Zinsser wrote that, in the chaos of the retreat

and Montreal, both of which lay in the path of westward-bound immigrants, suffered considerably. New arrivals from Europe brought the infection to Boston in 1838 and 1847, and to New York in 1818, 1825, 1837 and 1847. It was during the 1837 epidemic in Philadelphia that local physician William Wood Gerhard, who, while a medical student in Paris, had observed the distinctive intestinal lesions of typhoid, took medicine on its first major step toward distinguishing typhoid from typhus.

Throughout the early years of the 1860s typhus was 'remarkably frequent' in the eastern states, but nowhere to be found in the Mississippi Valley or the western states further testimony to the role of immigrants as carriers of the infection. Interestingly, however, neither the American Civil War (1861–5) nor the Franco-Prussian War (1870–71) spawned epidemic typhus, whereas the Eastern European revolutions of 1848, along with the Crimean War (1854–6) were typhus-ridden conflicts. This phenomenon underscores a shift of the geographical center of typhus to the east, to Russia, to the eastern portions of the Hapsburg Empire, and to the Ottoman Empire.

This retreat of typhus from the west to the east has been explained by the fact that there was social progress on one side of Europe and semi-medieval conditions on the other. But as the twentieth century got underway, medical science could claim some credit as well. In 1909 Charles Nicolle, director of the Institut Pasteur in Tunis, North Africa, showed that the body louse was to blame for spreading epidemic typhus, and, in 1910 Howard Taylor Ricketts, an American pathologist, discovered the pathogen which infected first the lice and then their human hosts. Ricketts died of typhus shortly thereafter,

Portrait of Howard Taylor Ricketts (1871–1910), a pioner in the study of rickettsial diseases, which are named after him. He died while investigating typhus in Mexico City.

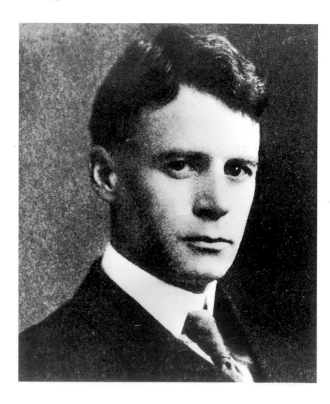

of 1916, the revolutions of 1917, and the onset of civil war, typhus alone caused the sickness of twenty-five million individuals under the control of the Soviet Union and the deaths of between two and a half and three million. Taking all the participants it has been estimated that during the war some thirty million people were infected with the disease of whom at least three million died.

In 1937 Herald R. Cox, of the US Public Health Service, discovered a method for culturing *rickettsiae*, which opened the way for vaccine production just as World War II loomed on the horizon. Concern about the threat that renewed typhus epidemics might pose for military operations led to the creation in 1942 of the USA Typhus Commission to battle the disease. The Cox vaccine was administered to all Allied military personnel and, although it was discovered that the vaccine did not really to prevent typhus, it did cause the illness to run a substantially milder course.

The fear of massive typhus outbreaks was clearly justified. Serious epidemics again appeared on the Eastern Front, in Yugoslavia, as well as in North Africa, Korea, Japan, Spain, Italy and Germany – especially in the concentration camps. Research, however, had proven the efficacy of an antilouse agent, DDT (dichlorodiphenyl-trichloroethane) which, as a powder, could be introduced under clothing by a 'blowing machine'. DDT dusting proved amazingly effective in combating a typhus epidemic in newly liberated Naples during the winter of 1943–4 and cut short other outbreaks in Germany that were ignited as concentration camps were liberated. The US government's concern for protecting its military personnel against typhus with the use of the Cox vaccine and DDT paid huge dividends. There were only 104 typhus cases in all of the Armed Forces and no deaths.

In 1947 it was discovered that broad spectrum antibiotics were effective against typhus and this, coupled with concerns about the side effects and the limited protection conferred by the Cox vaccine, ultimately led to its discontinuance. Another weapon against typhus was discarded when it was realized not only that DDT presented serious environmental hazards but that body lice were becoming resistant to it.

Since World War II, typhus has once again retreated to the poorer and cooler regions of the globe. It is reported most frequently from the Andean regions of South America, the Himalayan area in Asia, and the famine-ravaged horn of Africa. Zinsser joked that, because the lice always die from the typhus parasite, World War I had produced the greatest amount of lice mortality in the history of the world; and in the aftermath of World War II, DDT and antibiotics did them no good either.

Nevertheless, body lice are still very much alive and so is *R. prowazekii*. In fact, the pathogen survives in the tissues of patients even after they have recovered from the disease, only to resurface at a later time. This was first noticed by the physician Nathan Brill in 1898, among Hungarian Jews who had come to New York from an area where typhus had been epidemic. In 1934 Hans Zinsser hypothesized that this was a mechanism by which the disease could be carried over from one

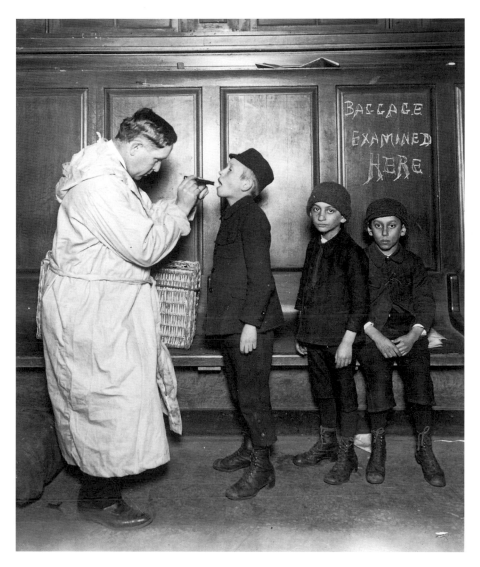

epidemic to ignite another – a hypothesis that was confirmed during laboratory investigations at Harvard Medical School in 1950–51. This form of the malady was named the Brill-Zinsser disease and serves as a reminder that typhus is a very tricky illness indeed.

Immigrant children newly arrived at the Battery from Ellis Island are examined by a New York City health official during a typhus scare in 1911.

BIBLIOGRAPHY

Ashburn, P. M. 1949. *The Ranks of Death*. Frank D. Ashburn (ed.). New York.

Harden, Victoria A. 1993. 'Typhus, Epidemic', in Kenneth F. Kiple (ed.), *The Cambridge World History of Human Disease*. Cambridge, England and New York.

Hirsch, August. 1883–6. 'Typhus', *Handbook of Geographical and Historical Pathology* (tr. Charles Creighton), 3 vols. London.

Kiple, Kenneth F. 1996. 'The History of Disease', in Roy Porter (ed.), *The Cambridge Illustrated History of Medicine*, pp. 16–51. Cambridge, England.

McGrew, Roderick E. 1985. 'Typhus', in Roderick E. McGrew (ed.), *Encyclopedia of Medical History*, pp. 350–55. New York.

Zinsser, Hans. 1934. *Rats, Lice, and History*. New York.

CHAPTER 17

SYPHILIS: THE GREAT POX

By Stephen V. Beck

Syphilis, a disease first noticed in Europe at the end of the fifteenth century, has been responsible for much physical suffering and death. In addition, social attitudes toward the victims of syphilis – at least in developed countries – have usually incorporated some degree of moral horror, with the result that a stigma has been attached to those afflicted by the disease.

Venereal syphilis is a sexually transmitted disease caused by a spirochetal bacterium, *Treponema pallidum*, of which humans appear to be the only natural host animal, and is thus one of the closely related group of diseases called the 'treponematoses'; the others are yaws, pinta and *bejel*, the Arabic word by which endemic or non-venereal syphilis is known. But whereas the other treponematoses are endemic to specific areas (for example, yaws – perhaps the oldest or most basic form of the infection – is generally restricted to the tropics), venereal syphilis has established itself across the globe and is in many places the most familiar of these maladies.

Syphilis has been called by many names. At first termed the 'disease of Naples', it soon became – both medically and popularly – *morbus gallicus*, the 'French pox' or 'French disease'. This was not the preferred term in France, and no fewer than six French medical writers of the sixteenth century attempted, without immediate success, to rename it. There is no doubt that sexually transmitted diseases had existed prior to this, although it is not clear whether they were recognized or classified as such. But the word 'venereal', taken from the name of Venus, the goddess of love, was first applied to syphilis in this period, and gradually the somewhat vague term 'venereal disease', referring to what we now regard as a number of separate symptoms caused by different pathogens, came into more or less general use. The Italian physician Girolamo Fracastoro, called by some the 'father of epidemiology', provided the name, 'syphilis', in his 1530 poem, 'Syphilis, Sive Morbus Gallicus', but this term was not much used before about the end of the eighteenth century. Up to that time, syphilis was also widely known as the 'great pox', thus differentiating it from the 'small pox', a name that we still use today for a quite different disease.

Modern research has revealed that the symptoms of syphilis develop through three phases, in between which the infection remains latent. These facts, however, were by no means clear to our forebears and, because of their inexperience with the disease, their symptoms were much more severe than those seen today. Our centuries of exposure have instilled a degree of tolerance – if not resistance – to syphilis that past humans did not enjoy.

In the first phase, the spirochetes enter the body (usually by penetrating mucous membranes) and incubate for about

Albrecht Dürer's The Syphilitic *(1496) graphically depicts the outward signs of the disease that horrified our forebears.*

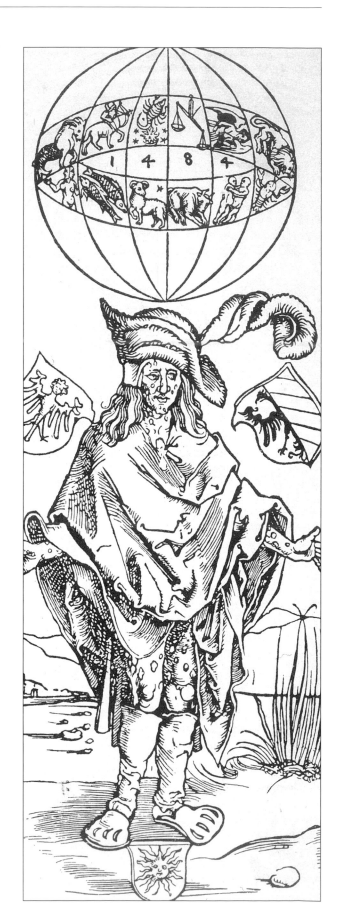

three weeks. Then, a small, painless lesion (or chancre) appears, most often at the point of entry. This seems to heal itself, disappearing after about a month, and a period of latency of several weeks ensues. In the second phase, multiple lesions appear on the skin and perhaps in internal organs as well. This rash is also painless, but is often accompanied by aches, fever and fatigue. Again, the symptoms of this phase vanish after a few weeks, but will recur in some victims.

Nowadays, only about one-third of untreated sufferers ever experience the third or 'late' phase of syphilis, and the latent period between the second and third phases may last for many years. In the late phase, the lesions may attack and destroy anywhere in the body, including internal organs and the skeleton as well as the skin. This phase is especially dangerous if the assault is mounted against the cardiovascular or central nervous systems. Although the records are not specific, it is logical to assume that this 'late' phase actually came earlier, and was even more pronounced, during the time when epidemic syphilis first struck Europe. In an inexperienced population, the sweeping destruction of bodily tissues may well have ensued immediately after infection and incubation.

Although syphilis is primarily a sexually transmitted disease, it can be contracted through direct contact with an open lesion. It can also be passed on to an unborn fetus by its pregnant mother, resulting in 'congenital syphilis', which may cause death or premature birth, or other complications.

Whether syphilis came to Europe from the Americas has been the subject of considerable debate. There are ancient Mesoamerican sculptures thought by some to represent victims of treponemal disease, as well as pre-Columbian skeletal remains with bone lesions that might indicate syphilis. In addition, early Spanish records of the New World note that the aboriginal Americans spoke of a syphilis-like disease as well known and well established, and the Spaniards themselves observed that the Indians seemed tolerant of it, possibly an indication of long acquaintance with the illness. It is sometimes difficult, however, to determine what disease was meant, as the Spanish term *bubas* or *bubos* was at different times used to mean syphilis, yaws, possibly another venereal disease, and even plague. Moreover, the presence in the New World of pinta – and possibly of yaws and some other unidentified treponemal infection – tends to confuse interpretations of the archaeological record.

Evidence is mounting that syphilis was present in Europe prior to 1492, but in a relatively mild form. This brings up the intriguing question of whether two treponemal diseases – one European and one American – fused to become the epidemic disease that burst spectacularly upon Europe at about the time that Christopher Columbus returned from his first voyage to the New World.

In 1493 and 1494 King Charles VIII of France conducted an ill-conceived invasion of Italy to wrest the kingdom of Naples from Spanish influence. As the two forces battled, an unfamiliar disease – the 'disease of Naples' – struck, causing casualties on both sides. But it waxed so virulent among the troops of the French king that he was forced to break off his offensive. His polyglot army disbanded, and, while returning to their respective homelands, the soldiers (including Britons, Germans, Hungarians and Poles, among others) scattered the infection – already being named the 'French disease', after the army that spread it – across the face of Europe.

Within a few years of these events, syphilis had become the most important endemic contagious disease in Europe. But it was more than merely endemic; soon, so many people were infected that syphilis seemed to be another plague, and, between 1493 and about 1530, Europe suffered a major epidemic of the 'new' disease.

Some Europeans noted quite early that the outbreak of epidemic syphilis had coincided with the return of Columbus from the New World, and certainly the pathogen appears to have behaved in Europe like a 'new' disease, at first raging among its victims and then decreasing in virulence as new generations were born. Such observations spawned the 'Columbian theory' of the disease's origin: that syphilis, endemic in the Americas and unknown in the Old World, had first been brought to Europe by Columbus's crewmen, albeit perhaps unwittingly, and had proceeded to wreak havoc upon a defenseless population.

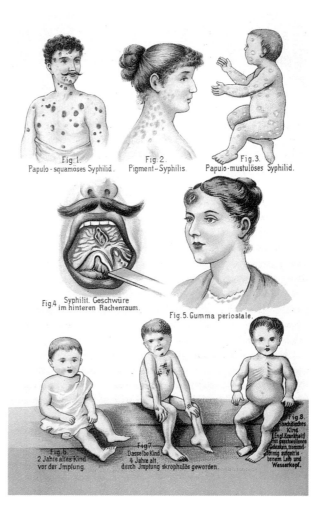

Chart giving a graphic representation of the various different indications of the condition of syphilis.

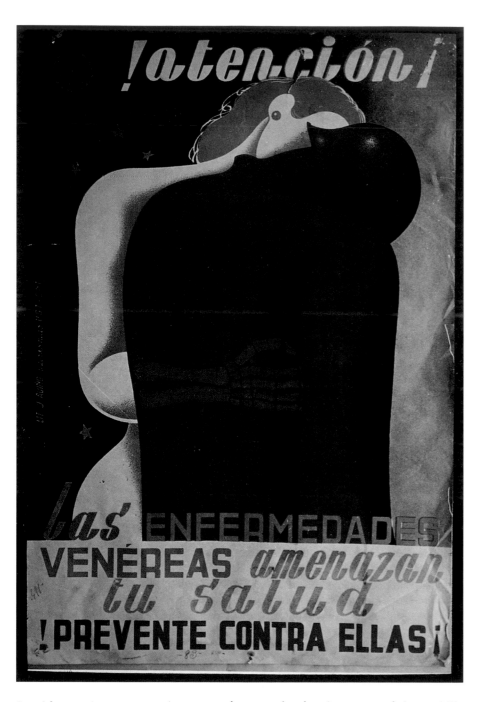

Spanish campaign poster warning of the risks of venereal disease and its fatal consequences.

syphilis and gonorrhea apparently resulted from different, or at least separate, conditions.

By the end of the eighteenth century, the rise of the middle classes created a new and harsher moral view of venereal disease. Now, having syphilis – by definition contracted through extramarital sexual intercourse – was irrefutable proof of immorality and symbolized vice itself. This not only meant personal disgrace for the syphilitic but an overwhelming social stigma as well.

In the nineteenth century medical research on syphilis, like the investigation of so many other diseases, at last began to be conducted in a systematic way. Partly as a result of Astruc's influence, the symptoms of venereal diseases were classified, distinctions were made between differing conditions and the terminology used to identify and discuss them was refined. Specialized works on specific venereal diseases appeared, as did specialized physicians and specialized hospitals. The French specialist Philippe Ricord, working at the Hôpital du Midi in Paris, created a large-scale program of research on venereal diseases, employing new chemical and technological techniques to perform thousands of experiments. In 1838 he reported that he had distinguished a specific syphilis 'virus' from other forms of venereal disease. In addition, he characterized the differences between primary- and secondary-stage symptoms and suggested a division of the stages similar to that in use today.

Ricord's ideas were refined as the nineteenth century progressed, and a number of distinct venereal diseases were identified. At first these were distinguished based on clinical evidence, but as the germ theory of disease gained the adherence of the medical profession, the individual bacteria were themselves discovered: the germ causing gonorrhea in 1879, and the bacillum that causes chancroid in 1889.

In the meantime, the study of syphilis was becoming an important field of research in medicine. The French specialist Jean-Alfred Fournier conceived the idea of the latent periods between the different phases of the disease and also proved that symptoms of bodily wasting, atrophy and paralysis were related to syphilitic infection. In 1893 he published a book on the treatment of the disease, but cautioned that there was no certain cure. Then, in 1905, German microbiologists Fritz Schaudinn and Erich Hoffman isolated *Treponema pallidum*, the syphilis germ and, the following year, the blood-serum test known as the Wassermann Reaction – for diagnosing syphilis through the identification of germs in a person's bloodstream – was invented.

An effective treatment for the illness, however, was still in the future. In 1928 British bacteriologist Alexander Fleming discovered the antibiotic penicillin. An unstable substance, penicillin was difficult to isolate and manufacture, but this was finally accomplished in the early 1940s, and before long the new antibiotic was found to be effective against all four of the human treponematoses, including syphilis.

times over subsequent decades. Astruc argued that syphilis and other illnesses were caused by particular 'viruses', and that these 'viruses' could be identified and categorized. Although in the light of present-day knowledge the author's theories and classifications seem rudimentary, they pointed toward the following century's development of the germ theory of disease, without which syphilis and many other infections might not have become treatable. Another important eighteenth-century book was *De Sedibus et Causis Morborum per Anatomen Indagatis* by the Italian anatomist and pathologist Giovanni Battista Morgagni, published in 1761, which presented his surgical discovery that the symptoms of

Despite the availability of such treatment, however, not all syphilis victims received it. It was revealed in 1972 that the US Public Health Service had for forty years been studying the course of syphilis in black men in Macon County, Alabama, without treating them. The 'Tuskegee Study' (named after the town where it took place) involved some 400 syphilitic patients who had applied for treatment, of whom perhaps one hundred had subsequently died. The fact that antibiotics had been available since the early 1940s only made this apparently racist research more incomprehensible, and ethical guidelines for human experimentation have been laid down as a result.

Since the development of diagnosis and treatment techniques for syphilis, the major advance in treponemal research has been theoretical. E. H. Hudson and C. J. Hackett, among other twentieth-century experts, have developed new ideas that attempt to account for the treponematoses as a group. Hackett has postulated that the differences among the diseases are the result of mutations by the spirochetes. Hudson, who first described *bejel* in 1928, has created the overarching 'Unitarian' theory.

Like the Columbian theory, the Unitarian theory is at once compelling and logical, but is based on evidence gained through the microscope and the laboratory: the spirochetes that cause the different treponemal diseases seem identical in both appearance and behavior. The Unitarian theory holds that these pathogens *are* identical, and that the different diseases – yaws, pinta, *bejel* and venereal syphilis – are the result of the same infection but are transmitted in different ways and manifest different symptoms under different climatic and cultural conditions. According to this theory, the treponemal spirochetes in Europe were perhaps just beginning to develop a sexual mode of transmission and the peculiar symptoms that accompany it at the end of the fifteenth century, and the return of Columbus's crewmen from the New World at about the same time was merely a coincidence.

From about the middle of the nineteenth century until the middle of the twentieth, syphilis incidence in developed countries declined, except in times of war, during which it has sharply, if briefly, increased. Since World War II, public health measures and the use of antibiotics have largely eliminated the incidence of both congenital syphilis and 'late' syphilis, but in recent decades the appearance of primary cases of the disease has increased again. In the last twenty years in the United States, it has been most common among people between fifteen and thirty-four years old. Males are almost three times as likely to contract syphilis as females, and male homosexuals are at extremely high risk; they account for half of all syphilitic men – a higher proportional incidence than for the rest of the male population. There also seems to be an increase in the number of syphilis cases in developing countries.

The upward trend in the appearance of primary-stage syphilis exists in spite of the most recent shift in society's moral view of the disease, beginning about the start of the twentieth century. This attitude depicts syphilis as not only immoral for the individual but, as a contagious and debilitating disease, dangerous to society. Consequently, developed countries have taken active steps, from legislating various compulsory public health measures to even declaring syphilis infection a crime. To contract syphilis is no longer an individual matter, whether of illness or morality.

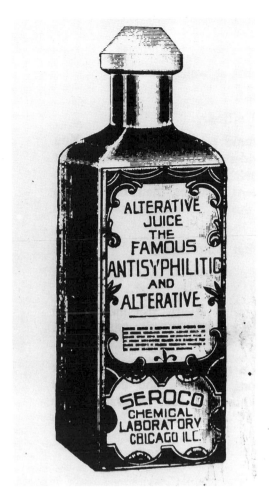

'Medicines' like 'Seroco' and other quack remedies and treatments have long been part of the history of syphilis and other diseases.

BIBLIOGRAPHY

Arrizabalaga, Jon. 1993. 'Syphilis', in Kenneth F. Kiple (ed.), *The Cambridge World History of Human Disease*. Cambridge, England and New York.
Hirsch, August. 1883–6. *Handbook of Geographical and Historical Pathology* (trans. Charles Creighton), 3 vols. London.
Quétel, Claude. 1990. *History of Syphilis* (trans. Judith Braddock and Brian Pike). Baltimore.
Temkin, Oswei. 1977. *The Double Face of Janus and Other Essays in the History of Medicine*. Baltimore.

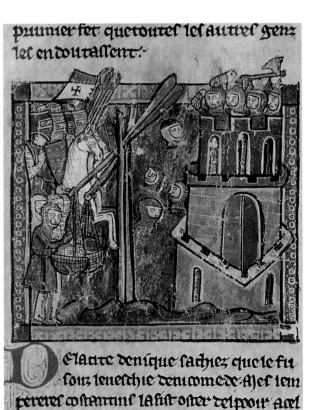

Crusaders bombard Nicaea with diseased heads in an early example of 'germ warfare', c. 1098. William of Tyre (c. 1130–85), Estoire d'Outremer.

PROGRESS, POVERTY AND PANDEMICS

As a rule, the complex social, economic, political and technological changes engendered by progress breed disease, and nowhere is this truer than in the history of pestilence in the eighteenth, nineteenth and early twentieth centuries. We regard the Industrial Revolution (and its continuation as a scientific, technological and information revolution) as an apex of progress, surpassed only by the Neolithic Revolution. But if the Neolithic Revolution, which stretched over thousands of years, produced towns and cities, rulers and ruled, and rich and poor, the Industrial Revolution did it all on a much greater scale and practically overnight. It spawned sprawling cities and massive poverty which led, for the first time, to widespread nutritional diseases.

The children of the urban poor in smoke-enshrouded urban and industrial centers grew up with the bowed legs and bossed skulls of rickets because of a lack of vitamin D. Peasants in southern Europe and mill workers in the southern United States suffered the dermatitis, dementia and death that pellagra brings because of such grinding poverty that niacin-deficient cornmeal made up the bulk of their diets. Steam-driven mills were invented to scrape away nutrients from other kinds of grains and especially the thiamine-rich husks and hulls of rice. The resulting white rice, although it stored well because it resisted spoilage, proved lethal to those whose poverty-dictated diets were based almost exclusively on that rice. Thiamine deficiency triggers the symptoms of both wet and dry beriberi to kill adults and passes through mothers' milk to kill their babies.

The progress represented by industrialization, urbanization and steam transportation also fostered the great pandemics of the nineteenth and early twentieth centuries. Indeed, without these innovations tuberculosis, cholera and influenza could not possibly have found their way to every corner of the earth. And, unfortunately, when they did, medicine was powerless against them. The incidence of tuberculosis, for example, was in dramatic decline long before means were devised to control it; the usual method of treating cholera patients by purging actually helped to kill the victims; and in 1918 vaccines against influenza were still in the future.

In the eighteenth and nineteenth centuries tuberculosis was more than anything else a product of urban poverty with the crowding, cramped quarters, poor nutrition, and the frequently appalling conditions of employment that accompanied it. In the twentieth century the industrial economies of the west seem to have helped to reduce the incidence of tuberculosis by providing, albeit grudgingly, the higher wages necessary for better housing and food. Where industrialization came somewhat later, as in Japan, tuberculosis mortality rates continued to soar during the first half of the twentieth century. In the case of tuberculosis, then, although progress can be blamed for creating favorable conditions for the disease to flourish, it should perhaps be credited with delivering the material benefits to lower tuberculosis mortality and morbidity, even taking into account that those populations caught up in the initial onslaught of the disease would have developed and passed on immunities to succeeding generations whatever their living standards.

Cholera, too, was a disease of poor sanitary conditions. Its cradle was the Ganges Delta of India where it had been confined for some 2,000 years. But in the nineteenth century that confinement ended, and the illness engulfed the globe in six rampaging pandemics. Once again, it was progress that had produced the steamships and railroads that could whisk cholera pathogens from city to city, and port to port, with a speed never before possible.

Progress was also implicated in the global cholera pandemics in other, less obvious, ways. The disease moves along the oral-fecal route, with water a favorite medium for reaching new victims. Although common water supplies for urban populations were hardly new (as the still standing Roman aqueducts testify), nineteenth-century urbanization spurred public and private efforts to provide rapidly growing populations with huge amounts of water from reservoirs, rivers, lakes and ponds. Unfortunately, this was considerably before knowledge developed of sanitation procedures that could insure the safety of that water. Thus, millions of people were at risk from cholera in the nineteenth century, who had not been at risk before and have not been since.

Then, too, in the nineteenth century the New World was increasingly a magnet for Old World immigrants, lured by the prospect of personal betterment. Packed tightly below the decks of ships in the most deplorable of sanitary conditions, their bodies frequently nursed cholera

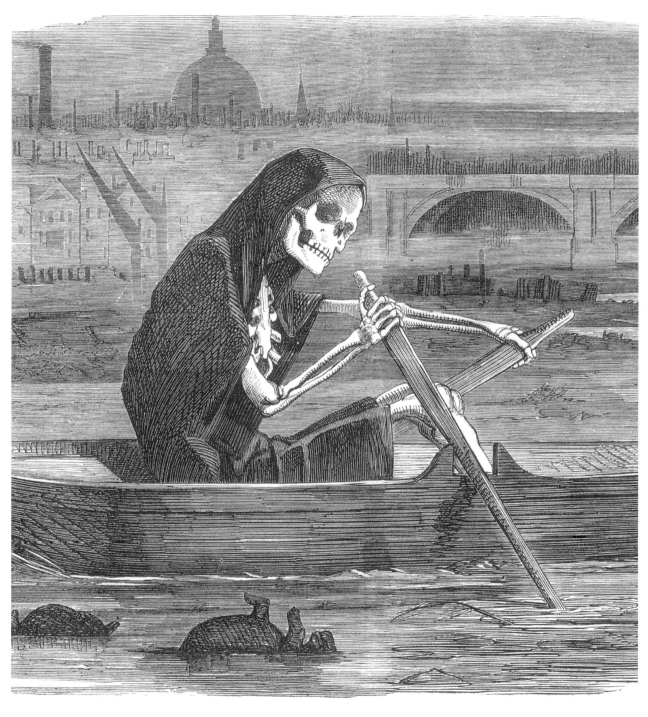

'The Silent Highwayman.
– Your MONEY or your
LIFE.' Cartoon Punch
magazine, 10 July 1858.

pathogens across the Atlantic to fall on populations in raging epidemics from Canada to Argentina.

The railroads and steamships had scarcely finished abetting the spread of cholera when they began to propel influenza around the world in the epidemic of 1918–19. This was an awesome epidemic that killed far more than the twenty-one million individuals that until recently were believed to have perished. Now we know that this number was based on incomplete data from many countries and that global influenza mortality was significantly higher. This epidemic may well have been the greatest single blow that pathogens ever unleashed on human hosts. Plague, cholera, tuberculosis, smallpox, typhus – all of the great, wide-ranging epidemics of the past – may have killed more people and greater percentages of populations, but they took years, even decades, to do it. The influenza of 1918–19 claimed the lives of perhaps as many as thirty million individuals in roughly six months. By striking contrast, deaths from all causes sustained by the armies of both sides during the four years of World War I which had just ended were estimated at eight and a half million.

Cultivation of maize and preparation of pancakes. Painted by Diego Rivera (1886–1957)

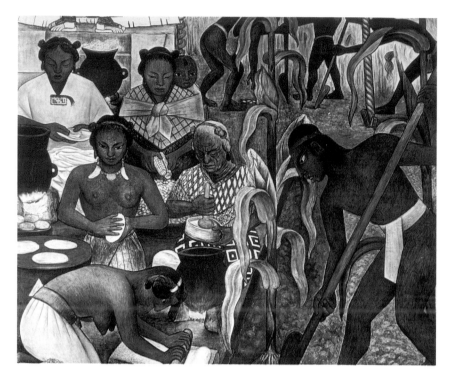

France had not been badly afflicted as yet, but, by the 1820s, the disease was beginning to take hold and arouse the interest of the medical profession there. In the meantime, little had been heard of pellagra in Spain since the publication of Casal's work. In the 1840s French physician Théophile Roussel conducted an investigation of conditions in Spain and, despite the objections of the Spanish medical men, published his conclusion that a number of illnesses then plaguing that country, although differently named, were all, in fact, pellagra.

Roussel became not only a medical expert on pellagra but also an advocate for social and economic changes that would help combat the disease. He wrote two books on pellagra that appeared in 1845 and 1866; these repeated Casal's observations that the illness had a dietary origin and was closely associated with maize consumption. Roussel argued for reforms in the national diet and food supply and in the economic conditions of the poor. The French government eventually responded by cutting back on maize production and encouraging the cultivation of other crops and an increased reliance on animal foods. As a result of these measures, pellagra was virtually eliminated in France by the end of the century.

Unfortunately, although Roussel saw the connection between pellagra and poverty, he also believed that it was the consumption of toxins in *moldy* maize grain that actually caused the disease. Despite some talk of nutritional deficiencies in maize, many influential experts, including several important Italian physicians, shared this view, which tended to obscure the important role played by people's

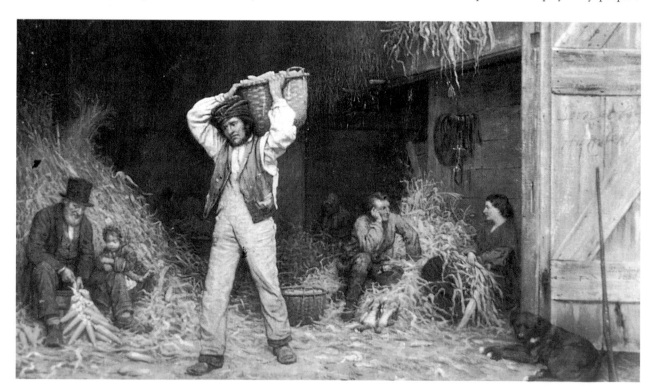

Corn-husking in the USA.

economic status. Such men were called Zeists after the botanical name of the maize plant, *zea mays*. During the rest of the nineteenth century their position received some degree of support from the obvious success of the French agricultural reforms and from recurrent outbreaks of pellagra – such as those in Yucatan, Mexico, in the 1880s and 1890s, and again from 1901 to 1909 – all allegedly the result of eating spoiled maize.

While European physicians attempted to deal with pellagra in their own countries, they were unaware that the disease was running rampant in other parts of the world as well. During the 1890s, however, British epidemiologist Fleming Sandwith, working in Cairo, Egypt, realized that pellagra was endemic in that region and began a systematic study of it. Echoing his predecessors, he found that pellagra was associated with a maize-based diet and extreme poverty (he added that residence in rural areas and exposure to the sun also seemed to be factors) and voiced agreement with the Zeist view that consumption of spoiled maize was the primary cause.

By his findings on endemic pellagra in Egypt, and the similar results of his study of the Bantu people in South Africa during the Boer War, Sandwith had shown that pellagra was by no means a strictly European problem; in fact, at the end of the nineteenth century, it seemed obvious that the disease had much greater footholds elsewhere. His discovery was a significant accomplishment, but perhaps an even greater one was that, through his reports and publications on pellagra (the first important ones to be written in English), he helped create awareness of it among American physicians, who were unwittingly faced with a pellagra problem of their own and would soon take the lead in fighting the disease. In the course of his researches into the geography of pellagra, Sandwith had corresponded with a number of medical men in the United States, but the disease seemed unknown to them. In fact, as we now know, it had been for some time almost epidemic in that country, especially in the American South. Pellagra had been rife among black people during the period of slavery and, after emancipation, among the southern poor generally. But it was often confused with other diseases and improperly diagnosed.

Like other nutritional deficiency diseases, pellagra often struck people in institutions – prisons, hospitals and the like – because the diet in such places was traditionally monotonous and restricted. An early example of this had occurred in 1817 in Italy, when two-thirds of the patients in a Milanese mental asylum were found to be suffering from pellagra. In addition, two of the earliest known cases in the United States, both reported in 1864, were patients in insane asylums, and pellagra was suspected as one of the chief causes of high mortality among Union soldiers in the Andersonville, Georgia, prisoner-of-war camp during the Civil War.

A number of other cases – perhaps even localized epidemics – appear to have occurred in the United States in the latter half of the nineteenth century. These were mostly among institutionalized people, but in many instances were poorly documented or misdiagnosed; certainly the medical

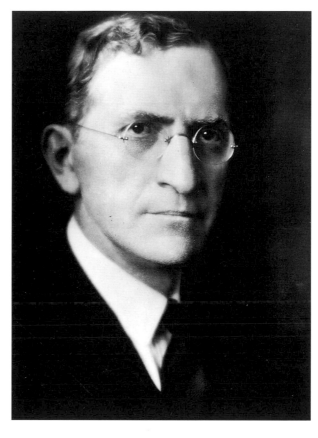

Joseph Goldberger, who initiated a multi-year study of pellagra that revealed that poverty and lack of dietary variety were consistently associated with the disease in the American South.

profession of the time took little notice of them. But in 1906 a pellagra epidemic broke out in the Alabama Institution for Negroes, a mental hospital, with shocking results: of the eighty-eight people affected, fifty-seven died. Unlike previous incidents, this catastrophe received a measure of publicity; in addition, it is thought that the doctors at the institution were not as ignorant of pellagra as so many of their colleagues elsewhere. Whether or not this was the case, the epidemic was fully reported and described in medical journals in 1907, and American physicians began to give the disease their attention. In subsequent months thousands of cases of pellagra were diagnosed, many of them in the southern states.

In spite of the general consensus of former times that pellagra had a dietary cause, other causes were now sought. Louis Sambon, of the London School of Tropical Medicine, put forward the theory that the disease was an infection delivered by an insect vector, the *Simulium* fly, functioning like the recently discovered insect vectors of yellow fever and malaria. The Zeist view, too, was still heard, and further confused the issue by proclaiming an incorrect dietary cause – moldy maize. Other groups blamed other foods.

New 'cures' for pellagra abounded. Despite debatable effectiveness and danger to their patients, physicians made liberal use of 'Fowler's solution', 'Atoxyl', 'Salvarsan' and other arsenical preparations. They also employed purges, antiseptic injections, various tonics, blood transfusions from recovered pellagrins, and, in one case, 'treatment' with static

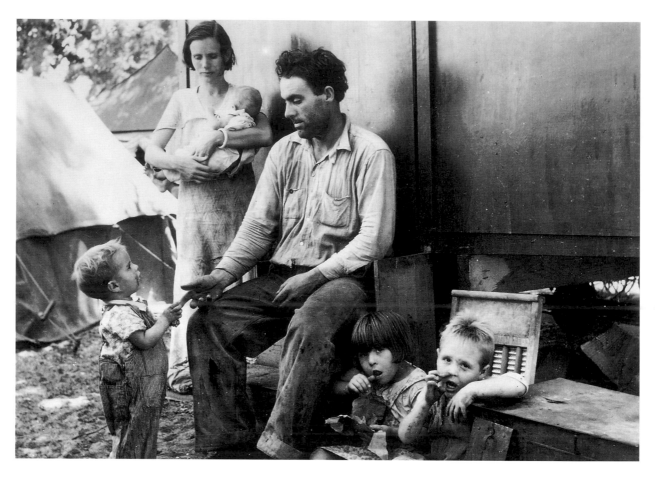

electricity. A US congressman referred to the latter cure as 'simply marvelous'.

Also much in evidence were patent medicines and 'quack' remedies, such as 'Ez-X-Ba River, The Stream of Life', sold for five dollars a bottle by the Dedmond Remedy Company, founded in 1911 by Ezxba Dedmond. This product was reputed to cure pellagra within weeks, and early in its history the company claimed hundreds of cures. Another quack product was 'Pellagracide', made by the National Pellagra Remedy Company. Both South Carolina-based firms were challenged in 1912 by that state's Board of Health and denounced as fraudulent by the American Medical Association – analysis of the concoctions revealed no active elements at all – but they remained in business. In 1913 'Doctor' Baughn's American Compounding Company followed much the same course with its 'Baughn's Pellagra Remedy' in Alabama. The quack medicines enjoyed much more popularity and confidence among the general public than did the treatments offered by legitimate physicians; indeed, the first encounter many poor pellagra victims had with a doctor was when they were already near death and committed to a mental hospital.

Following the epidemic in Alabama, the US Public Health Service entered the battle against pellagra, and, beginning in 1914, the Service's Joseph Goldberger succeeded in curing institutionalized pellagrins by altering their diets. His next

trial, also successful, was to induce the disease in prison inmates who volunteered to subsist on a restricted diet. In addition, he proved through experiments on himself and his colleagues that pellagra was neither transmittable nor infectious.

Goldberger initiated a multi-year study of the disease that revealed that poverty and lack of dietary variety were consistently associated with pellagra in the American South. The study, which later attained renown as a classic model of epidemiology, showed conclusively that pellagrous mill-workers and agricultural laborers were on the lowest rung of the economic ladder, and that the traditional diet of the southern poor – cornmeal bread, 'fat-back' pork and molasses – was all that most of them had access to, or could afford. Poverty, manifesting itself through bad nutrition, had resulted in pellagra attaining epidemic proportions among the lowest-paid in society.

Goldberger had proved that the cause of pellagra was a dietary deficiency caused by the prevailing social and economic conditions. Further tests indicated that the diet of pellagrins lacked a crucial element, referred to as the pellagra-preventing factor (the 'P-P factor' for short), and that this substance, though yet unidentified, was present in meat and dairy foods and some vegetables.

Goldberger would spend the rest of his life trying to identify the P-P factor. In the 1920s he went to work at the Hygienic Laboratory in Washington, DC, and soon learned that researchers at Yale University had identified 'black tongue' in dogs as analogous to pellagra in humans. Using dogs in dietary tests, Goldberger and his team accidentally discovered that yeast was a rich source of the P-P factor, although they still did not know what that elusive substance was. Nevertheless, at Goldberger's urging, yeast was distributed in 1927 to thousands of flood victims, specifically to avert pellagra. Following the great success of this operation, distribution of yeast became a common practice in cases of disaster and in poor relief during the Great Depression.

Goldberger died in 1929 after having found another source of the P-P factor in animal livers, but he never knew what the substance was. Pellagra, still a major health problem in the United States at that time, began to decline during the Depression as government programs and economic pressures forced agricultural diversification and increased the quantity and general quality of the food supply, especially in the South. Finally, in 1937, Conrad A. Elvehjem and colleagues at the University of Wisconsin identified the P-P factor as niacin, also known as nicotinic acid. Niacin treatment of pellagrins was tried out on a large scale in hospitals – and it worked.

Since then, pellagra has vanished from many places where it was once endemic; its occurrence nowadays, even in areas where it remains a problem, is more likely to be endemic rather than epidemic in nature. In recent years the disease has been connected with diets based on millet or sorghum grains as well as those based on maize. These other grains contain niacin in an unbound form, which can be absorbed by the body, but also contain relatively high amounts of the amino acid leucine, and it is believed that the presence of excessive leucine causes an imbalance of amino acids and contributes to niacin deficiency. These grains commonly constitute a large proportion of the diet of agricultural workers in places such as Egypt and the Indian subcontinent, where pellagra continues to appear. The disease is also still associated in the modern world with famine, and has recently afflicted people in famine-stricken areas of Africa.

In developed countries the near-disappearance of pellagra is as much the result of changing social and economic conditions – largely a rising standard of living – as it is of medical advances and improvements in public health and nutrition, although the wider availability of a variety of vitamin-enriched foods has made a significant difference. It can, however, still be seen in some developed countries in connection with alcoholism, which is one of a number of indications that the biochemical changes underlying both the physical and mental symptoms of pellagra have yet to give up all their secrets to medical researchers.

BIBLIOGRAPHY

Beardsley, Edward H. 1987. *A History of Neglect: Health Care for Blacks and Mill Workers in the Twentieth-Century South.* Knoxville.
Etheridge, Elizabeth W. 1993. 'Pellagra', in Kenneth F. Kiple (ed.), *The Cambridge World History of Human Disease.* Cambridge, England and New York.
Hirsch, August. *1883–6. Handbook of Geographical and Historical Pathology* (trans. Charles Creighton), 3 vols. London.
Kiple, Kenneth F. and Virginia H. Kiple. 1977. 'Black Tongue and Black Men: Pellagra and Slavery in the Antebellum South', *The Journal of Southern History* 43, pp. 411–28.
Roe, Daphne A. 1973. *A Plague of Corn: The Social History of Pellagra.* Ithaca, New York.

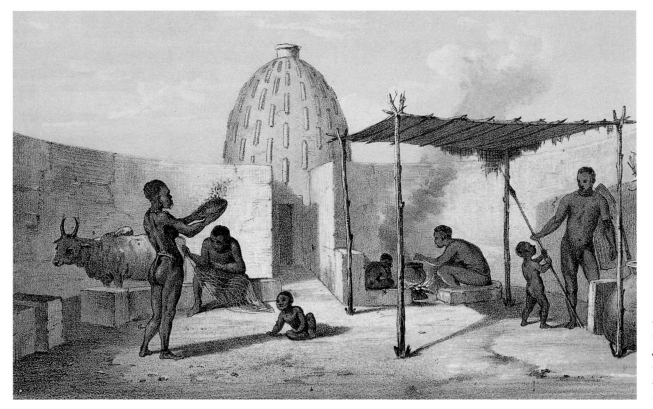

Interior of Musgu dwelling near Chad, showing a grain storage bin. Sketch by Dr Barth from his travels and discoveries in north and central Africa.

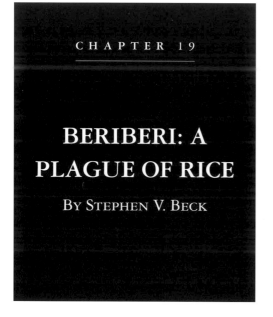

CHAPTER 19

BERIBERI: A PLAGUE OF RICE

By Stephen V. Beck

Beriberi, once a mysterious, deadly illness that is now generally curable, has probably killed millions of people through the ages. Also called *kakke* or *ashike* in parts of East Asia, it has been known as a specific disease entity in China and Japan since ancient historical times. It is mentioned in one of the oldest medical texts known in human history, a Chinese work dating from more than 4,000 years ago. When Europeans reached East Asia during the 'Age of Exploration', they must have encountered and identified the condition quite soon. Early seventeenth-century records – from the Spaniards in the Philippines and the Dutch in the East Indies – contain a number of references to beriberi, although the first published description of it by a European is attributed to the Dutch physician Jacob Bontius in 1645. The origin of the word 'beriberi' itself has been disputed. It is often said to come from a Sinhalese word that means 'weakness', but it may also have derived from the Malay word for 'sheep' – apparently because the disease can make people walk in a peculiar sheep-like fashion.

The symptoms of beriberi vary, but include nerve problems (lack of feeling and, in advanced or extreme cases, paralysis), loss of strength or energy, an enlarged heart, palpitations, abnormally low blood pressure, and swelling of the face and limbs. As a result of the diversity in symptoms, several types of beriberi have been distinguished. 'Dry beriberi' tends to involve mainly the central nervous system, moving from loss of sensation and motor control through paralysis and muscular atrophy, whereas 'wet beriberi' generally produces cardiac symptoms along with swellings and fever. An acute, heart-threatening form of the disease has been named '*shoshin* beriberi'. Finally, there is 'infantile beriberi', occurring in unweaned infants, with symptoms like those of wet beriberi but also including digestive problems or other symptoms not seen in adult beriberi cases. Severe cases of beriberi, even if treated or cured, may result in mental illnesses such as Wernicke's encephalopathy and Korsakoff's psychosis, and all forms of the disease may, if untreated, result in death.

The cause of beriberi was not known with certainty before the twentieth century, but in the past it was ascribed to, among other things, low-lying regions, the weather or the season, spoiled food, poisoning by various organic or inorganic chemicals, or infection by known or unknown germs. By the end of the nineteenth century a few researchers were beginning to suspect that the condition was brought about by some nutritional deficiency. Nowadays we know that all forms of beriberi are the result of a deficiency of thiamine (also known in the past as vitamin B_1) in the human diet.

Thiamine is essential for the proper metabolism of food by all living things. It is especially vital in converting carbohydrates and sugars into energy for the body, and also helps to metabolize amino acids, which make up proteins. A number of different foods contain thiamine. Yeast, whole grains, various kinds of beans, liver and kidneys, and oysters all have relatively high amounts; it can also be found in pork and many green vegetables. One reason why the symptoms of beriberi are so varied and complicated is that deficiencies of different vitamins often go hand-in-hand. A thiamine deficiency in the diet commonly indicates that other B vitamins are lacking as well; for example, modern medical thinking now inclines to the belief that the symptoms of dry beriberi involve riboflavin (vitamin B_2) deficiency in addition to that of thiamine.

Nowadays, people who may be at risk for beriberi include pregnant women and their unweaned children, kidney-dialysis patients, and persons who are fed intravenously for long periods. More generally, people who use a great deal of energy, that is, laborers or anyone consistently performing hard physical work, may be at risk if their diet is thiamine-deficient. In addition, it was realized not long ago that the disease poses a significant threat to alcoholics. Alcoholism leads to a reduced ability of the body to absorb thiamine and at the same time increases its need for it. Moreover, an alcoholic may fail to consume a wide variety of foods. Taken

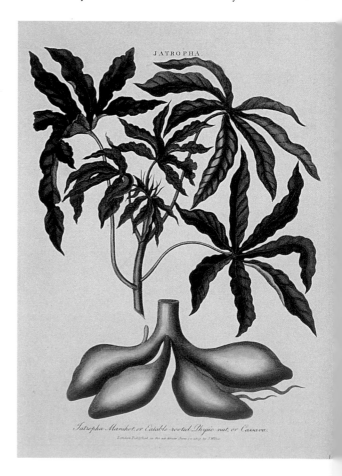

JATROPHA

Jatropha Manihot, or Eatable rooted Physic-nut, or Cassava.

Cassava or tapioca plant.

together these factors can result in beriberi complicated by mental illness and problems of the nervous system.

Historically, particular categories of humans have been extremely susceptible to beriberi. People in institutions – such as mental hospitals or prisons – or on board ships have typically subsisted on diets that lacked variety, much like the situation experienced by sufferers from scurvy. In the eighteenth and nineteenth centuries beriberi was common among Brazilian laborers and slaves, whose diet was limited mainly to dried meat and manioc (cassava) flour, both foods with extremely low thiamine content. Most significantly, beriberi has been closely associated with rice-subsistent populations. Where rice makes up the bulk of the food that people eat (accounting for perhaps 80 percent of the total calory intake), de-hulling the grain can effectively eliminate thiamine from the diet because virtually all the thiamine is contained in the grain's outer husk, or hull. Thus, although the disease has historically struck various population groups worldwide, it is the Asians, whose staple food is rice, who have suffered most.

Humans require an intake of only a few micrograms of thiamine each day, and de-hulling rice by hand probably leaves enough bits of the hull (the 'bran') in the grain to satisfy a person's thiamine requirements. But, with the advent of modern industry, de-hulling and 'polishing' of rice came to be done in mechanical rice mills, which removed almost all the bran and, as a result, nearly all the thiamine.

Another dietary factor related to thiamine deficiency is the enzyme thiaminase, which is found in raw fish (among other foods) and reacts against thiamine. Usually beriberi results from a diet deficient in thiamine, but it can also be caused or worsened by a diet heavy in foods with thiaminase. For example, in Laos and northern Thailand rice is steamed, which helps preserve its thiamine component. But the people of this area eat a great deal of raw fish paste, the high thiaminase content of which can wipe out the thiamine in the diet and thus produce beriberi.

Asian food preparation techniques have also affected the nutritive value of rice. Thiamine can be eliminated by excessive washing of the grain, as was long the custom in Japan, whereas in many parts of Southeast Asia the custom of cooking rice with too much water removes the vitamin from the diet. On the other hand, in India and Sri Lanka, as in Laos, the custom of parboiling or steaming rice prior to the milling process has been effective in preserving the thiamine in the grain, even when it is de-hulled and polished, and these countries, despite a sizable consumption of rice, are on the whole relatively free of beriberi. But this practice has failed to catch on in most other rice-eating parts of Asia.

During the nineteenth century beriberi epidemics struck sailors on ships in many different parts of the world. North Atlantic fishing fleets were hard hit, as was the Brazilian navy. Outbreaks were frequent among all shipping in an arc stretching around Asia from the Sea of Japan to the Bay of Bengal. 'Ship beriberi' was thought at one time to be a somewhat different illness from other forms of beriberi because it afflicted the crewmen of western ships, whereas in other circumstances most victims seemed likely to be Asians. A related theory postulated that beriberi was contagious among Asians. On land, however, the disease attacked inmates of institutions and military personnel throughout much of the world, from prisons and asylums in the United States to troop garrisons in the Congo.

Beriberi was long associated with proximity to large bodies of water, such as oceans or rivers, and also with a tropical climate and wet weather. During the second half of the nineteenth century, in Brazil, Burma, India and Japan, the disease, which had formerly been thought to belong to the sea coasts, began moving inland; this seemed to indicate that locality and climate were not primary causative factors. In fact, the apparent inland march of beriberi was actually a movement from urban to rural areas as the disease followed the spread of over-milled, polished rice. This was an early result of the development of mechanical rice mills, which were first built in large cities (many of which were coastal ports) and only later in more remote locations along transportation routes.

All sorts and classes of people contracted beriberi, so that differences in various social and public-health practices could be discounted as causes of the disease. It was also noticed that people newly arrived in beriberi-stricken areas – for example,

JASIONE AND JASMINUM.

1. Hairy Sheep's Scabious. 2. Common Jasmine, with the caterpillar of the Sphinx atropos, or Jasmine Hawk-moth, feeding on it.

was probably not distinguished from other deforming skeletal conditions, and with many of the passing references to such illnesses that we have, it is difficult to determine what specific disease – if any – is being described.

Rickets received more detailed attention from medical scholars in the seventeenth century. An early work was the Dutchman Daniel Whistler's *On the Disease of English Children Which Is Popularly Termed the Rickets*, published in Latin in 1645. This was soon followed, in 1650, by Englishman Francis Glisson's *De Rachitide* (On Rickets), which many have called the classic description of the disease. Another Britisher, John Mayow (also known for other scientific and medical writings) published his own *On Rickets* in 1668. Both Glisson and Mayow emphasized that it was a disease of infants and young children. Although rickets has no doubt existed as long as humans have, all three of these writers believed that the condition had only arisen very recently, even within their own century. Mayow, for example, suggested that rickets had first appeared in western England around the 1620s, and had since spread throughout the country.

If the disease was endemic, it is difficult to believe that its high incidence had not been observed in previous times. On the other hand, if there was an 'epidemic' of rickets in this period, there must have been a reason for it. Some have speculated that it might have reached epidemic proportions because of recent developments in social conditions; it also seems possible that relatively long-term climatic changes could have affected its prevalence.

Glisson and Mayow differed, however, over the cause of the disease. Glisson speculated that the characteristic curvature of the long bones might be caused by them receiving more nourishment, and thus growing more, on one side of the bone than on the other. Mayow disagreed with this, stating that the cause was unrelated to nourishment of the bones: they grew anyway, but the attached muscles failed to receive sufficient nourishment, failed to grow, and by remaining too short restricted the straight growth of the bones.

Making allowances for the state of their knowledge of nutrition and biochemistry, these scholars were on something like

Liverpool Docks, by John Atkinson Grimshaw (1836–93). The blotting out of sunshine by smoke and smog led to a substantial increase in rickets incidence in industrializing countries.

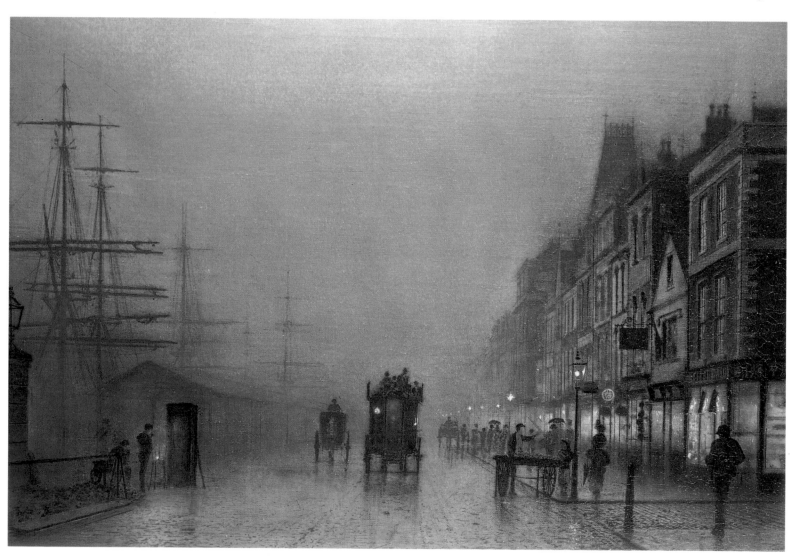

the right track in their analysis of the causes of rickets. But the cures they proposed were nothing to inspire confidence, consisting as they did of enemas, purgatives and diuretics, inducement of vomiting or sweating, bloodletting (with leeches), tapping of spinal fluid, bathing in hot springs, exercise (which could have been quite painful), vigorous massage with woolen cloths or various ointments or plasters, splints and bandages, whalebone corsets, and the use of a device like a sort of portable traction harness.

Their treatises helped to focus the collective medical mind on rickets, but more than a century passed before any real advance was made, until in the late eighteenth century cod-liver oil was found to be effective against the disease. Thomas Percival, a physician in Manchester, England, in 1789 discussed the properties and benefits of this rather unpleasant substance, now known to be a generally rich source of vitamin D (though the level of its vitamin content is variable). But it would be more than another hundred years before the vitamin itself was discovered, and in the meantime, little progress was made against a disease that was assuming epidemic proportions.

In the late eighteenth century and throughout much of the nineteenth, the Industrial Revolution, with its palls of coal smoke and smog screening out ultraviolet rays, and its crowded, unlovely, urban ghettoes blotting out sunlight altogether, led to a substantial increase in rickets incidence in industrializing countries. Working-class children in British industrial cities of this period may have gone for weeks, even months, at a time without the necessary exposure to sunlight. Charles Dickens's character, the crippled 'Tiny Tim' from *A Christmas Carol*, was probably meant to be understood as a rachitic child. In fact, rickets was known to some as the 'English disease'.

But rickets was hardly confined to England or even to Europe. According to historical and scientific evidence, it is likely that the disease prevailed among slaves in the United States. Mortality statistics on black children and newspaper advertisements describing the personal appearance of runaway slaves indicated both a great number of people with rickets-like symptoms and an unusually high incidence of the most severe types of cases. Many American physicians came to believe that such data proved an innate vulnerability to the disease on the part of black people.

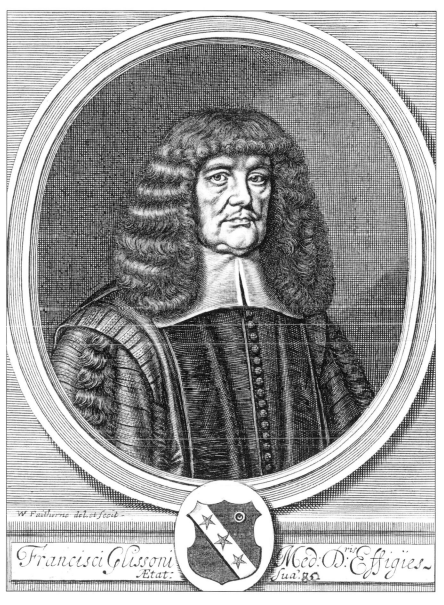

W Faithorne del et fecit

Francisci Glissoni Ætat: Med: D:ris Effigies Sua. 85

In 1650, English scholar Francis Glisson published the classic De Rachitide *(On Rickets). Despite the rudimentary medical knowledge of the period, Glisson postulated that the disease arose from a nutritional problem.*

But it was shown in the 1960s that the various skin pigmentations of humans affect the process of vitamin D synthesis. Black skin absorbs only a third as much ultraviolet light as white skin, so that, when the blacks were forcibly removed from their tropical, sunny African environment to the more overcast temperate zone, they became substantially more rickets-prone.

The tendency of blacks in North America to develop rickets remained high even after their emancipation from slavery, and in the early twentieth century – when much more was known about the disease, and the discovery of vitamin D itself was imminent – researchers announced their fear that as many as 90 percent of black children in the United States might suffer from it. It has been reported that, even some decades later in the 1950s, the rate of deformed pelvises among black women was seven and a half times (15 percent vs. 2 percent) that of white women.

Fumigating passengers from Marseilles to Avignon.

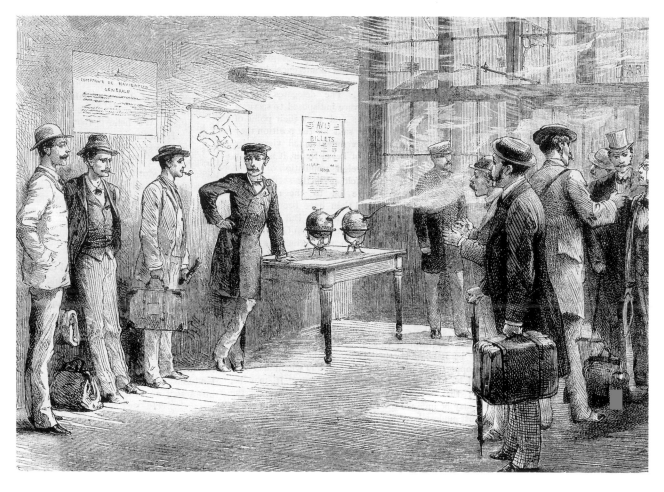

indictment of wealth and luxury and unwonted pride. Witnessing the epidemic in Paris, the young German poet Heinrich Heine described cholera at a carnival party; his words were then transformed by Alfred Rethel into the memorable image of death appearing among the revelers, playing a femur and tibia as a violin. Across the Atlantic, Edgar Allan Poe read of the cholera and wrote his 'Masque of the Red Death'.

As suddenly as cholera came, it disappeared. Documented failures of quarantine stimulated medical doubts about the contagion model and reinforced theories of the environmental and moral predisposing factors that made cholera favor the poor and improvident more than the clean, godly and prudent. But in the decade after cholera's first assault on the West, urban poverty and urban squalor continued to expand. Unfortunately the gospel of sanitation was no less costly than that of quarantine.

In 1854 a Florentine microscopist, Filippo Pacini, first clearly described the cholera vibrio, drawing upon autopsy studies of victims. Also in that year John Snow, a young, teetotal, vegetarian physician working in one of the shabbiest quarters of Dickensian London, tested his hypothesis that cholera was waterborne by studying the household spread of cases. Snow seems to have been the first to use 'spot' maps to chart the local spread of cholera, marking every cholera death

in the area around the public pump on Broad Street on a simple street map. He interviewed the families of each new cholera case, determining where they obtained their drinking and washing water, and persuaded the aldermen to remove the pump's handle on 7 September 1854, two weeks after the local epidemic began. But typical of cholera epidemics, whatever their magnitude, these two weeks had allowed the

CHOLER ...

THE
DUDLEY BOARD OF HEALTH,

HEREBY GIVE NOTICE, THAT IN CONSEQUENCE OF THE

Church-yards at Dudley

Being so full, no one who has died of the **CHOLERA** will be permitted to be buried after *SUNDAY* next, (To-morrow) in either of the Burial Grounds of *St. Thomas's,* or *St. Edmund's,* in this Town.

All Persons who die from CHOLERA, must for the future be buried in the Church-yard at Nethertor

BOARD of HEALTH, DUDLEY.

At the height of the cholera epidemics in the 1860s, it was believed that infected corpses would contaminate the soil and contribute to the spread of cholera.

disease to run its course; the murderous phase of the epidemic was over.

Snow's claims were fairly well known in Great Britain and North America, but London governors were convinced that they could repel cholera simply by tracking its geographical spread from Hamburg, Germany westward, and then taking last-minute measures. New York sanitarians, on the other hand, used Snow's information to take swift and impressive control of cholera in 1866. Without any costly investment in cleaning up slums, clean water could be supplied for a limited time period and the houses of victims disinfected. Thus, in the English-speaking world cholera was conquerable by 1860, without any specific knowledge of its cause and without clear understanding of effective therapy.

Meanwhile, Max von Pettenkofer, a Munich hygienist and sanitarian, reasoned from the erratic incidence of cholera infection that both the bodies of the infected and the soil of the cities had to contribute an essential factor if cholera were to take hold. Some soils, he believed, lacked the factor that unleashed cholera's power. Moreover, he thought that chemical conditions — heat, motion, aeration, for example – also affected the outcome. For Pettenkofer far more than for Snow, understanding the causal nexus was essential to scientific intervention. Pettenkofer's sophisticated and detailed attention to the chemical components of urban water supplies, to the procedures of large-scale water purification and analysis, and to the general management of environmental toxins and effluvia had far greater influence on the anti-choleric practices of later nineteenth-century Europe than did Snow's shoestring analysis of a few hundred cholera cases in London.

An international sanitary conference was set up in 1851 with the express intent of controlling incursions of cholera. Most of these gatherings – twelve occurred before World War 1 – convened to address new appearances of cholera. International public health objectives were muted during the 1860s, 1870s and early 1880s, however, because many of the principal European powers were at war with each other, and little consensus about international controls evolved. Moreover, frightening as cholera epidemics were, official concern was somewhat muted because mortality tended to peak among the very poorest urban dwellers. In addition, continued bickering among medical scientists about the cause and transmission of cholera also served to attenuate and deflect pan-European objectives for international sanitary controls.

News of cholera in Alexandria in 1883 provoked the French and German governments to dispatch investigating teams to the scene. Louis Pasteur was then over sixty years old and frail, so he sent two of his prized assistants, Emile Roux and Louis Thuillier, as part of the four-man French team to Alexandria. Roux, Thuillier and two pathologists arrived in mid-August when the epidemic was already in precipitate decline, but they zeroed in on evidence from autopsies, including preliminary results of microbial cultures from the blood, stool and guts of cholera victims. In their reports,

however, they made the understandable mistake of concentrating on the victims of cholera. Tragically, Thuillier died of the disease.

Robert Koch, the founder of German bacteriology, also investigated the outbreak of cholera in Alexandria. His eventual success rested on his pursuit of two different lines of investigation. He understood the importance of studying the individual microorganism and its relationship to disease. A

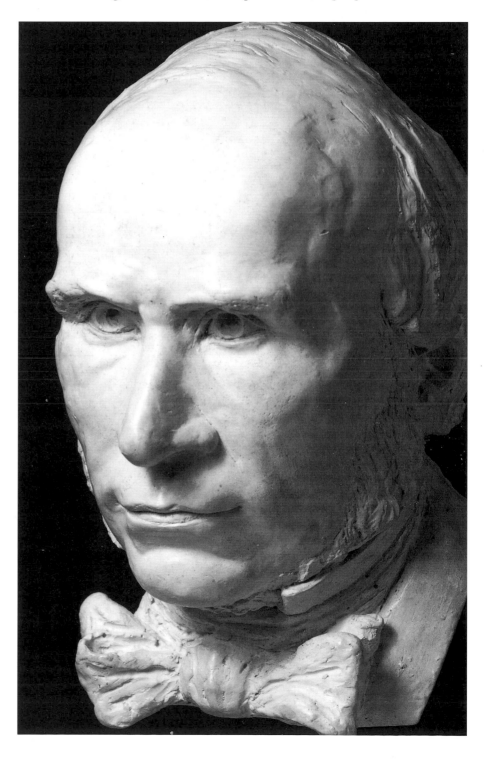

Plaster cast bust of John Snow, who in 1854, convinced that cholera was waterborne, persuaded the aldermen to remove the handle of the Broad Street pump.

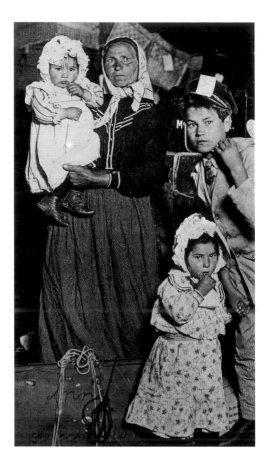

A refugee family at Ellis Island, fleeing cholera.

Cartoonists in the earlier nineteenth century ridiculed physicians' inability to cure cholera. Patients were urged to protect themselves in so many ways that, outfitted for cholera prevention, their garb was comical.

focus on the germ itself, its life cycle, its nutritional requirements, its distinctive morphology, and its particular environment ensuring optimal growth, had led Koch to attend to tedious laboratory details. Pasteur's trainees were still using liquid (broth) culture media that could poorly separate the many different intestinal organisms; Koch had already developed solid media on which to grow bacteria. His overall methodology placed his team at an advantage.

Running out of 'fresh' victims, he was also eager to pursue an itinerary that led back to cholera's source. Because his team arrived late in Alexandria and because he could not succeed in infecting any of the experimental animals he brought with him or found (Koch even tried to inoculate crocodiles and ibises), they traveled south to the German East African port of Dar es-Salaam and headed east. He knew at this point that the intestines of people who died of decidedly non-choleric diseases never contained the vibrio, and that those of cholera victims did. But he could not prove that the vibrio was the cause, rather than a consequence, of the disease. So he began to focus on the *absence* of cholera in the absence of the vibrio. Koch demonstrated that no cases of cholera occurred when the vibrio organism was not present.

From December 1883 until the heat of April 1884 shut down his makeshift laboratory, Koch focused simultaneously on obtaining pure cultures of the vibrio microbe, on searching for a suitable experimental animal among the fauna of Southeast Asia and on making careful notation of where and in whom cases of cholera appeared, as well as where it failed to appear. His team rushed to the sites of small, focal outbreaks of cholera in the teeming suburbs of Calcutta, where water tanks looking more like ponds lay in close proximity to clusters of cholera cases, and the distinctive comma bacillus was in the communal water supply. But where there was no vibrio, there was no

cholera. Koch had essentially replicated the epidemiological insights of John Snow, whose work he did not know. He returned to Berlin on 2 May 1884, triumphant.

Ironically, cholera traveled to Europe again not only in the cultures of the vibrio that Koch carried back, but along the same familiar routes. The French ports of Toulon and Marseille were infected by June 1884, and a concerted cover-up by local officials permitted the spread of cholera to other, unsuspecting Mediterranean ports. Of these Naples was a prime target. The city was squalid beyond the tolerance of most other Italian cities because its élite were blind to the abject poverty of immigrants from the countryside. Cholera quickly destroyed 7,000 Neapolitan lives, even though over 150,000 people had fled. In the aftermath the government of the newly united Italy turned extraordinary resources to the reconstruction – the *risanimento* or sanitizing – of the city, but the program was ultimately defeated by corruption and inertia.

Traveling overland, cholera took longer to reach northern Europe, but by 1891–2 it had returned to Moscow, and from there followed Jewish immigrants fleeing persecution. Many trains headed for Hamburg and Bremen, where large ocean liners offered the refugees cheap passage to Britain and North America. If cholera reached Russia, Hamburg was certain to see it too. Robert Koch, now head of the Prussian Imperial Health Office and more confident of his cholera facts than any man alive, issued orders for the epidemic's control,

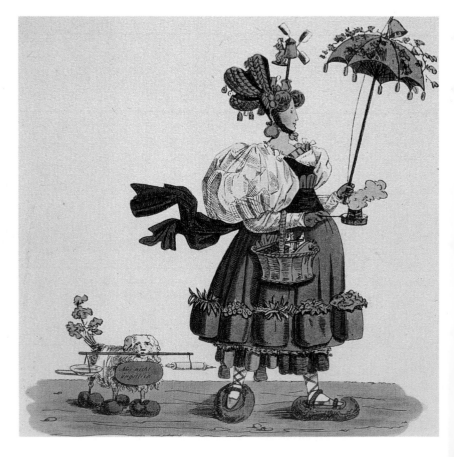

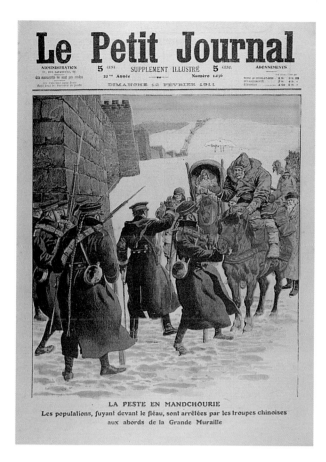

LA PESTE EN MANDCHOURIE
Les populations, fuyant devant le fléau, sont arrêtées par les troupes chinoises aux abords de la Grande Muraille

elegance and simplicity of Koch's explanation of cholera closed the door to arguments about predisposing factors and conditions.

Cholera in the early twentieth century was quickly repositioned as a disease that Muslim pilgrims occasionally carried out of Asia. Soon after the turn of the century, Egypt's El Tor quarantine station began to see pilgrims to Mecca with very mild cases of cholera, the earliest instances of the less virulent strain of cholera typical across the world today. Since the 1960s the 'El Tor' strain of cholera has been quite successful, far better at reproducing itself than its classic, virulent relative. The story of cholera is thus an unfinished one.

BIBLIOGRAPHY

Arnold, David. 1993. *Colonizing the Body: State Medicine and Epidemic Disease in Nineteenth-Century India*. Berkeley, California, and London.

Coleman, William. 1987. 'Koch's comma bacillus: the first year', *Bulletin of the History of Medicine* 61, pp.315–42.

Delaporte, François. 1986. *Disease and Civilization* (trans. Arthur Goldhammer). Cambridge, Massachusetts and London.

Evans, Richard J. 1987. *Death in Hamburg: Society and Politics in the Cholera Years, 1830–1910*. New York and London.

Howard-Jones, Norman. 1975. *The Scientific Background of the International Sanitary Conferences, 1851–1938*. Geneva.

Snowden, Frank M. 1996 *Naples in the Time of Cholera: 1884–1911*. Cambridge and London.

Cover of Le Petit Journal, *1911. 'The Plague of Manchuria: the population fleeing from the plague, are stopped by the Chinese troops on the borders of the Great Wall.'*

sealing the borders to the east. Hamburg's respondents, however, appealed to the evidence of multiple causative factors still argued by von Pettenkofer – the Hamburg élite had not accepted the premise that government had a financial responsibility for general public health surveillance beyond protecting the lives, properties and prospects of its governing citizens. During the 1860s and 1870s other cities – including Altona immediately across the Weser River from Hamburg – had invested in water purification systems, and because they did so, they were spared; Hamburg's governors had instead decided that the responsibility for purifying drinking water lay with individual property owners. Maximizing profits, entrepreneurs in this fierce capitalist enclave eschewed costly regulation of housing, and even failed to monitor health conditions in the temporary quarters for refugees passing through. The workers' accommodations, or 'Alley Quarters', near the city's shipping center were like an oily rag ready for the flame of cholera. When Koch made an official visit to the stricken, squalid areas, he ungloved his exasperation with Hamburg's public officials. His indictment made international news: 'Gentlemen, I forget that I am in Europe.'

Max von Pettenkofer, whose soil-contamination theory of cholera's spread was still upheld by many, stubbornly resisted the simple idea that a bacillus could cause a phenomenon as unpredictable as cholera in its choice of individual victims or epidemic sites. But by the 1890s the

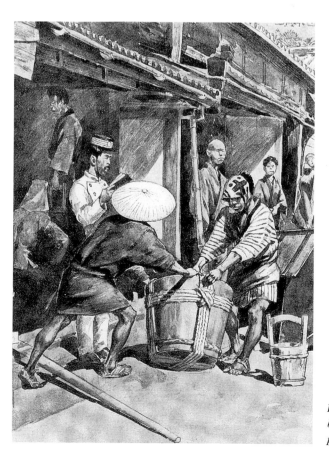

Disposing of the dead in barrels, under police protection, Japan.

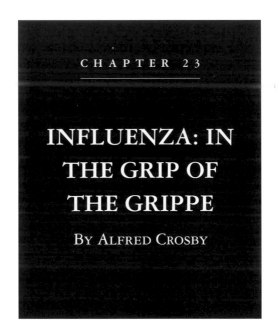

CHAPTER 23

INFLUENZA: IN THE GRIP OF THE GRIPPE

BY ALFRED CROSBY

'Good Evening. I'm the new influenza.' An influenza cartoon by Ernest Noble, 1918.

Influenza is a sly, nimble, ambiguous, deceptive sort of disease. Sometimes, usually during the warmer months, no one seems to have it, and sometimes, usually during the colder months, everyone seems to have it. It spreads by breath and has an incubation period of only one to two days, so it often seems to strike a whole population at once. In the last 200 years it has several times rolled around the whole world, north and south, east and west, in a year or less, putting hundreds of millions in bed and sometimes infecting the majority of our species at least sub-clinically (symptomlessly). Eighteenth-century Italians explained its seemingly universal effect by deciding that it must be the product of astrological conditions, of the universal influence of the stars, so they named it 'influence', *influenza*.

Flu, as it is often called (or grippe, as the French have named it) hits fast with sore throat, cough, runny nose, fever, chills, headache, aching muscles and joints, and a yearning to go to bed and stay there. Short of resorting to laboratory analysis of sputum, the best way to differentiate between influenza and a bad cold, with which it shares so many symptoms, is by checking on the disease's prevalence. If a whole lot of people are prostrated with respiratory illness at once, then it is probably influenza.

In the great majority of cases flu victims are miserable for no more than a week or so. There may be two or three more days of feeling below par, and then the patient is back to normal. There seem to be no lasting effects, but there were many cases of brain inflammation (*encephalitis lethargica*), an affliction superficially quite unlike respiratory influenza, in the 1920s, which probably were a final Parthian swipe of the great 1918–19 flu pandemic.

In all but a few years the death rate of flu is 1 percent or less, and almost all the dead are among the very young or the very old. But – and this is why influenza can be called sly – it infects so very many that the small percentage who die amount, in absolute numbers, to a lot of people. And when this infection opens the path for bacterial pneumonia, it is a killer. In the United States in the 1980s influenza, when paired with pneumonia, was one of the ten leading causes of death. Yet if most people were asked to list the diseases they feared most, few would even think of that old excuse for going to bed for a week and having people look after you, the flu.

Another reason for calling it sly is that a bout of influenza, unlike one of measles or mumps, produces only short-lived immunity. You can, and many of us know this from unpleasant experience, get influenza again and again. That is why within a human generation flu can repeatedly roll around the globe, shifting with the sun from northern to southern hemispheres and back. And there is no cure. You have to wear it out or it wears you out.

We share many diseases with our primate cousins, but influenza is not one of them. It is unlikely that such a swiftly communicable illness existed among our hunter-gatherer ancestors, because they lived in small groups, in which the disease would have infected everyone fast and either killed them or temporarily immunized them. That is to say, it would have burned out and disappeared.

Ancient medical texts are often incomplete in coverage and ambiguous in their clinical descriptions and doubtlessly have nothing to say about any number of infections in circulation 1,000, 2,000 or more years ago. However, one would think that an epidemic of influenza would have been so spectacular that Hippocrates, for instance, would not have omitted it from his writings. The first unequivocal description of a flu epidemic is an account of the epidemic of 1510.

As for where the disease started, one can only guess. The comparatively high death rates of flu sufferers among the Amerindians, Australians and other peoples outside of Europe, Asia and Africa suggest that it has probably existed longest in the Old World continents. The fact that it is an infection we humans share back and forth with domesticated animals, such as pigs and fowl, suggests that it has existed longest in parts of the world where people have had herds and flocks of such animals longest. That would, again, be in the

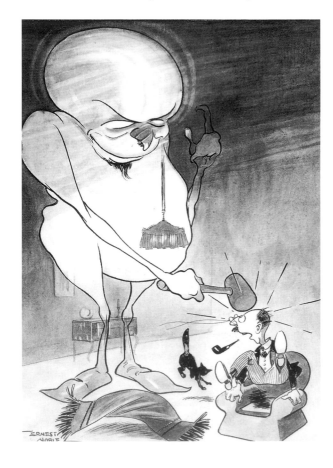

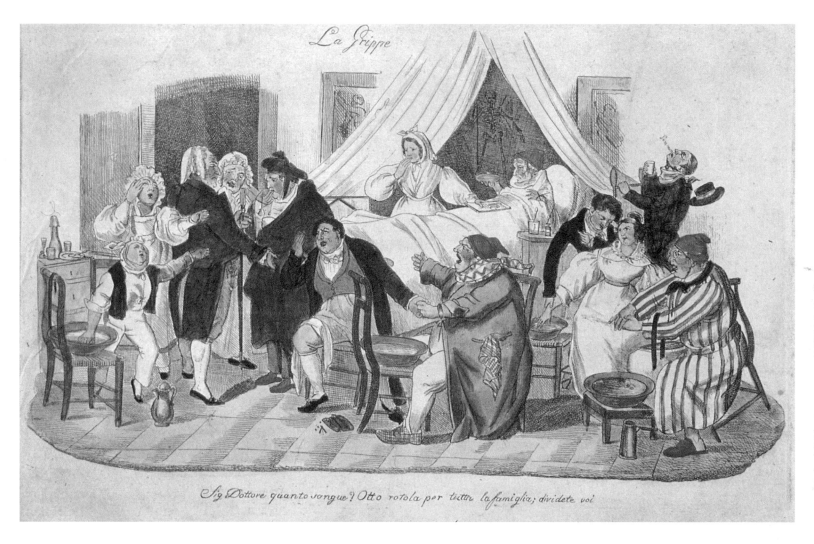

La Grippe

Sig Dottore quanto sangue? Otto rotola per tutta la famiglia; dividete voi

Old World. But humans also share the disease with undomesticated birds.

The educated guess as to flu's geographical origin is that it started in the Old World. If so, then it is another of the terrible gifts of pathogens that European mariners, merchants and colonists carried with them across the oceans to the epidemiological innocents who lived beyond.

There were three epidemics of influenza in Europe in the sixteenth century: 1510, 1557 and 1580. The last of these rolled from the Mediterranean to the Baltic in four months and deserves the title of pandemic. The seventeenth century was a time of relative inactivity for influenza, at least in Europe. There were regional outbreaks, but no pandemics. In the eighteenth century, as human populations, especially urban ones, began to increase rapidly along with herds and flocks, influenza resumed its role as a spectacularly communicable infection. There were at least three and possibly as many as five flu pandemics in Europe in the 1700s, plus regional epidemics. The worst of them all was that of 1781–2, which started in the east and swept over Europe, where it was called 'la Russe' and 'catarro russo', and spread on to the Americas. It made tens of millions ill and killed many

of them. It was the most impressive of the early examples of what population growth and improving transportation systems could do in extending the reach of influenza.

In the nineteenth century there were at least three more such pandemics, in 1830–31, 1833, and 1889–90, and a number of regional epidemics. In the last epidemic when, again, it entered Europe from the east, the disease was called Russian flu. It swept Europe in December of 1889, crossed the Atlantic and appeared in North America in the same month. It spread widely in all the populated continents and reached New Zealand, which was as far away from the pandemic's alleged point of origin as one could get. It killed an estimated quarter of a million people in Europe and several times that in the world, but the proportion of the dead, expressed as a percentage of the ill, was very low, and most of the dead were very young or very old, so influenza still maintained its false reputation for gentleness.

For the last decade of the nineteenth and first seventeen years of the twentieth century the flu sputtered but did not explode, despite increasing speed and frequency in transportation and despite the violence and malnutrition caused by wars and rebellions in South Africa, China, Russia,

A family threatened by influenza undergo bleeding.

'Doctors giving Thanks to Influenza', by James West, 1803.

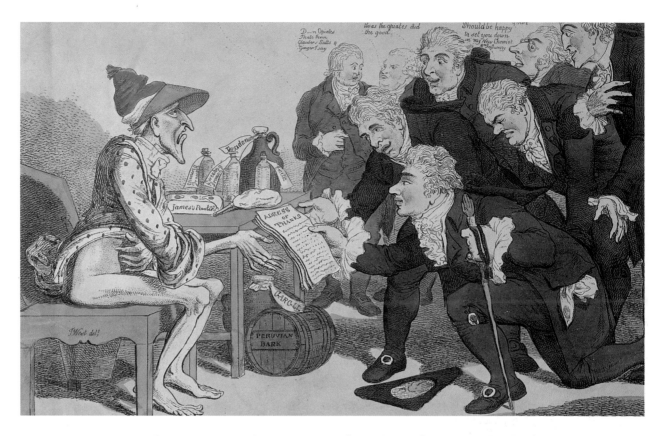

etc., mounting to a crescendo which culminated in the chaos of World War I. Then, in the late winter or early spring of 1918, possibly beginning in the United States, which the great war only touched indirectly, a wave of the usual kind of 'mild' influenza rose, and in the summer swept over the world. It killed few; its only distinctive quality, not noticed till later, was that an oddly large proportion of the few who died in the spring and summer were young adults.

By the end of summer the pandemic faded, having spent itself. But in the latter part of August the virus changed, turning into the deadliest of its kind of all time. The odds are enormously in favor of its having done so in one place and then spread out from there, but the fact is that it first surfaced almost simultaneously in three places far distant from each other: Boston, Massachusetts, in America; Freeport in Sierra Leone on the coast of West Africa; and Brest, the port of Brittany, France. All three were ports engaged in gathering and dispatching troops and supplies from all over the world to the trenches of the Western Front. There is no evidence that this virulent influenza virus was the result of the 'crossing' of viruses from disparate geographical sources, but it is tempting to harbor that thought.

The tidal wave of influenza in the fall of 1918, supplemented by a third and lesser wave in the winter of the following year, was unprecedented and not repeated since, but not necessarily because it infected so many. Records compiled at the time indicated that millions upon millions fell ill; and blood tests carried out later showed that it touched the majority of the human race. But it is conceivable that the

flu pandemic of 1889–90 and those of the second half of the twentieth century may have infected as large a proportion of the population. The 1918 flu had two unquestionably distinctive characteristics. Firstly, it killed not only the young and the old, but those in the prime of life: about half the

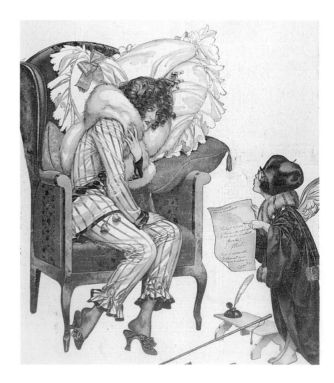

'Suffering from Spanish flu', at the time of the Armistice (1918).

victims were between twenty and forty years of age. Secondly, it had a distinctive propensity for itself initiating pneumonia or encouraging bacterial secondary infections to do so. In ten months it killed at least 550,000 citizens of the United States, about ten times as many as had died in combat in the war. The mortality in India in October 1918 was 'without parallel in the history of disease', according to one official. The demographer Kingsley Davis has suggested that 20 million may have died in India alone. The pandemic did its worst in Western Samoa, where 7,542 died out of a population of 38,302 in November and December 1918.

The first careful estimate of the number of flu deaths in the world, made in the 1920s, set the figure at 21 million. Scholarly re-examination of the records since has raised the estimate to 30 million. The influenza virus of the autumn of 1918 and winter of 1919 killed more people than World War I and more people than anything else in history in the brief period of one year or less. World War II killed a greater number, but took five years to do so.

The flu catastrophe of 1918 attracted more attention to the disease than ever before. Scientists worked for years with enormous handicaps: they couldn't see the villain, the flu

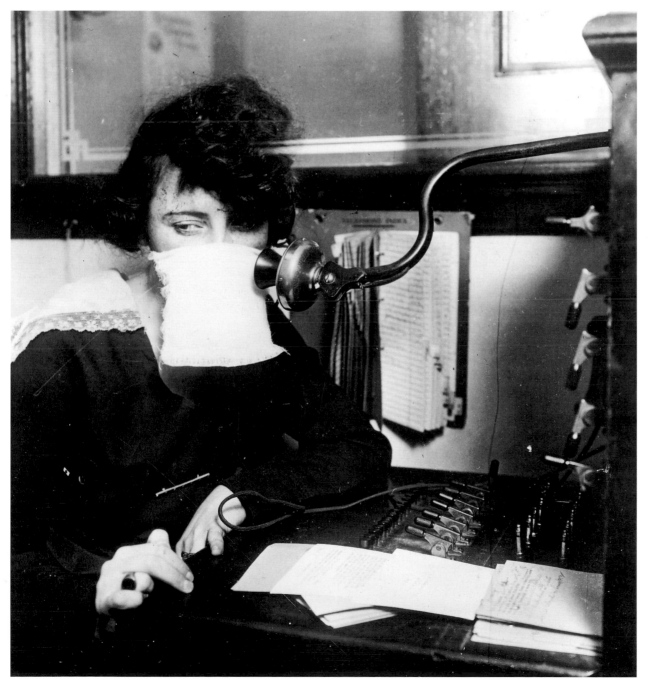

A telephone operator with a protective mask in 1918.

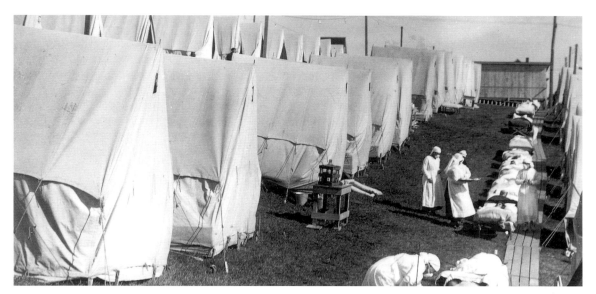

Tents for influenza cases, Canada.

Then, in about 1930, the American Richard E. Shope was able to transfer an influenza-like disease from a sick pig to a healthy one via a liquid obtained from the former from which everything visible had been filtered. In Great Britain researchers discovered that the ferret could get flu and, though a nasty beast, could be worked with in the laboratory. They succeeded in giving the animal human influenza via a clear filtrate. (One of the scientists then caught flu himself from a sneezing ferret – perhaps not a carefully controlled experiment, but one which confirmed that they were working with human influenza.)

virus, with the kind of microscopes that they had in the 1920s; they had no guinea pigs, white rats or any other laboratory animal to work with because, as far as was known, flu was strictly a human infection. There was no real progress for years.

In the 1930s scientists utilized the new electron microscope to see and photograph the influenza viruses. There are three categories: A, B and C. B and C cause mild illnesses and don't spread pandemically. It is A that gives rise to acute illness and pandemics. It has a genetically unstable surface which alters constantly, if slowly, even during

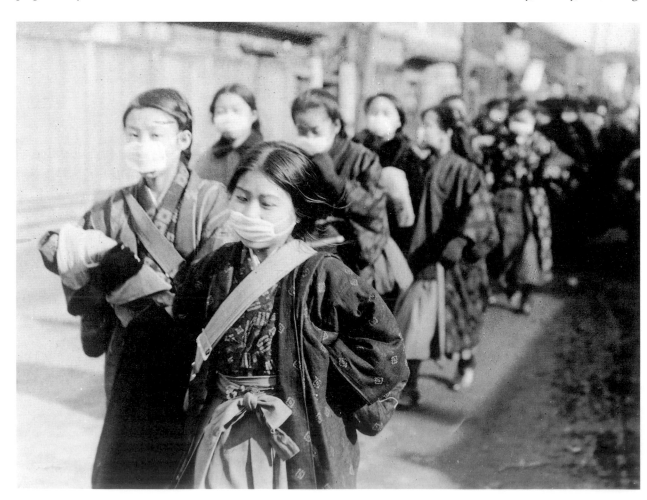

Japanese schoolgirls wear protective masks during the great influenza pandemic.

the period of the few weeks or months of a given epidemic, often frustrating the best efforts of physicians and virologists. Vaccines, first mass-produced in the 1940s, may be effective one flu season but not the next, and their usefulness the third year is decidedly questionable.

The outside surface of the flu virus changes radically several times a century. When that happens, as in 1918, 1957 and 1968, the majority of humans, whatever their previous contacts with influenza, are liable to infection, that is to say, a pandemic explodes. Our defenses against that swiftly moving disaster are vaccines, if they can be discovered, mass-produced and pumped into the arms of millions fast enough to dampen the pandemic's advance. Our reaction time has to be swift indeed because of our globe-spanning transportation systems: someone carrying a new flu from Ulan Bator may be deplaning at Heathrow at this very minute. Our ability to predict where the next dangerous flu strain will appear is enormously complicated by the fact that we share and exchange flu viruses with our domesticated mammals and birds and with wild creatures, as well. We may all be cooperatively engaged in cultivating new strains. The next influenza pandemic may hit us from, for instance, China, where people and pigs live in contiguity in thousands of villages, and where new strains of influenza virus may be spawning all the time. Or the next pandemic strain may appear in one of the richest, most medically advanced societies on the planet. Our best defense is our early-warning system of about a hundred centers around the world reporting new flu strains as they appear to the World Health Organization.

Early warning enables national public health organizations to develop suitable vaccines and to distribute them to the populations for which they are responsible. It also enables them to make expensive mistakes. In 1976 a few cases of what seemed in the laboratory to be a virus quite like that of the 1918 pandemic appeared in an army camp in New Jersey. The United States spent millions of dollars to produce a vaccine to save the world from a reprise of the 1918 catastrophe, vaccinated millions of its citizens against it – and there was no pandemic, not even an epidemic, associated with this strain of the virus. The best that President Ford and the American flu fighters could say was that it was better to have a vaccine and no pandemic than a pandemic and no vaccine.

Nowadays the situation is by no means grim, but not cheering either. Influenza viruses with the frightful characteristics of that of 1918 have not spread. Attempts to recover and revive viruses from cadavers of 1918 in an effort to learn what made them so dangerous continue to be made, and are beginning to pay off. That strain might come back with dreadful consequences, but it is also true that we might learn of its reappearance early enough to produce a relevant vaccine and distribute it. In addition, we now have antibiotics to control the secondary bacterial infections that were involved in the deaths of so many three-quarters of a century ago. Finally, our molecular biologists are working on medications undreamed of even twenty-five years ago. They haven't been tried on humans yet and what works on lab animals may not work on people, but there is hope that continued research and trials may eventually lead to a cure for influenza.

Scientists and public health experts have accomplished miracles in learning the habits of the influenza virus and the strengths and weaknesses of the human immune system vis-à-vis that tiny entity. It is a long way from the fall of 1918, when the following ditty circulated as undertakers worked day and night and the graveyards fillied up:

'I had a little bird
And its name was Enza.
I opened the window
And influenza.'

BIBLIOGRAPHY

Crosby, Alfred W. 1989. *America's Forgotten Pandemic: The Influenza of 1918*. Cambridge, England.
Dutton, Diane B. 1988. *Worse than the Disease: Pitfalls of Medical Progress*. Cambridge, England.
Kilbourne, Edwin D. 1987. *Influenza*. New York.
Patterson, K. David. 1986. *Pandemic Influenza, 1700–1900: A Study in Historical Epidemiology*. Totowa, New Jersey.
Phillips, H. 1990. *Black October: The Impact of the Spanish Influenza Epidemic of 1918 on South Africa*. Pretoria.
Rice, Geoffrey. 1988. *Black November: The 1918 Influenza Epidemic in New Zealand*. Wellington, New Zealand.

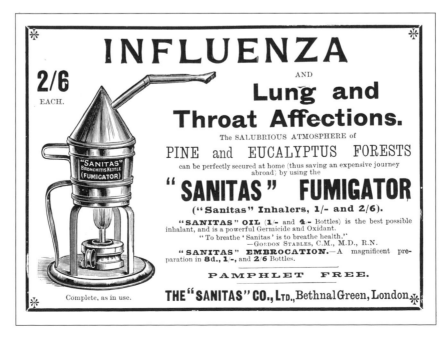

There are no cures for influenza, but we have always tried. 1900 advertisement in the Illustrated London News.

EPHEMERAL INFIRMITY

This final section of the book features some mysterious illnesses of the historical past that remain mysteries to this very day. We call them ephemeral because although at one time they were thought to be disease entities, today, for one reason or another, they are no longer with us and in many cases we can only speculate on what they might have been. Two examples, which are drawn from the many ephemeral diseases that we do not deal with in the following pages, are nonetheless interesting to cite because of the way in which they illustrate something of the range of reasons why diseases can become ephemeral. One is the famous Plague of Athens which took place close to two and a half millennia ago. In this instance the disease may be unrecognizable in the present because when it was described so long ago, it was in a stage ancestral to some illness we came to know much later in a very different stage of development. Whatever it was, the Plague of Athens has been credited with changing the course of history by abruptly bringing down the Athenian army and putting an end to Athenian imperialism.

A considerably more recent example concerns a disease which entered American medical textbooks during the last half of the nineteenth century. This illness was called typhomalarial fever, and it was thought to be a hybrid that combined elements of malaria, typhoid, and perhaps other diseases as well. Such a fusion was believed to be most likely to occur among closely congregated troops and it was regularly diagnosed among them from the American Civil War through America's war with Spain. But as it turned out, the disease was really only typhoid alone and as the famous Canadian physician and medical historian, William Osler, observed, typhomalarial fever seems to have 'existed in the minds of doctors but not in the bodies of patients'. If there is any mystery left for us today it is how a disease that did not exist could have been routinely diagnosed for over half a century.

Between evolving diseases such as the Plague of Athens and physician-created illnesses like typhomalarial fever

fall numerous other examples of ephemeral pestilence, three of which we do discuss in this section. One was the 'sweating sickness' which made a series of staccato-like assaults on the English that began at the end of the fifteenth century and continued to the middle of the following one, before (apparently) vanishing for ever. Equally intriguing is the fact that sweating sickness seemed to be attracted to just one group – the English – while leaving other groups – the Scots, the Welsh and the Irish – virtually unmolested.

The next illness under scrutiny is chlorosis, which was also called the 'green disease', because sufferers (almost all female) frequently took on a greenish pallor. Because of this apparently distinctive symptom some have been reluctant to dismiss chlorosis as just one more illness that existed more in the minds of doctors (and their patients) than in the bodies of patients. Moreover it has a lengthy history. Chlorosis was diagnosed as early as the time of Hippocrates, and flourished as a disease in the nineteenth century. But because it disappeared totally in the first two or three decades of the twentieth century the question arises as to what chlorosis really was. The answer seems to be that it was a number of conditions, or perhaps better, a cluster of symptoms that although once associated by physicians (who agreed there was a disease called chlorosis), became subsequently disassociated with better diagnostic techniques.

The last of our plagues, and in many ways the strangest, is a compulsion to dance. Tarantism – a disease of women in the region of Apulia in southeast Italy – was thought to be caused by the bite of a tarantula and to be curable by wild dancing – the spider's dance – to regional music. Such curing has been going on at least since the Middle Ages, leading some to suspect that the tarantulas in that region are unique. Most, however, have dismissed the phenomenon as a product of superstitious minds. Nevertheless tarantism has survived the Scientific Revolution, the Age of Enlightenment, and the medical advances of both the nineteenth and twentieth centuries. Cases still appear in Apulia, even today.

Hunterian Psalter. Hunter 364 (top V14 f.59). John Bannister delivering an anatomy lesson.

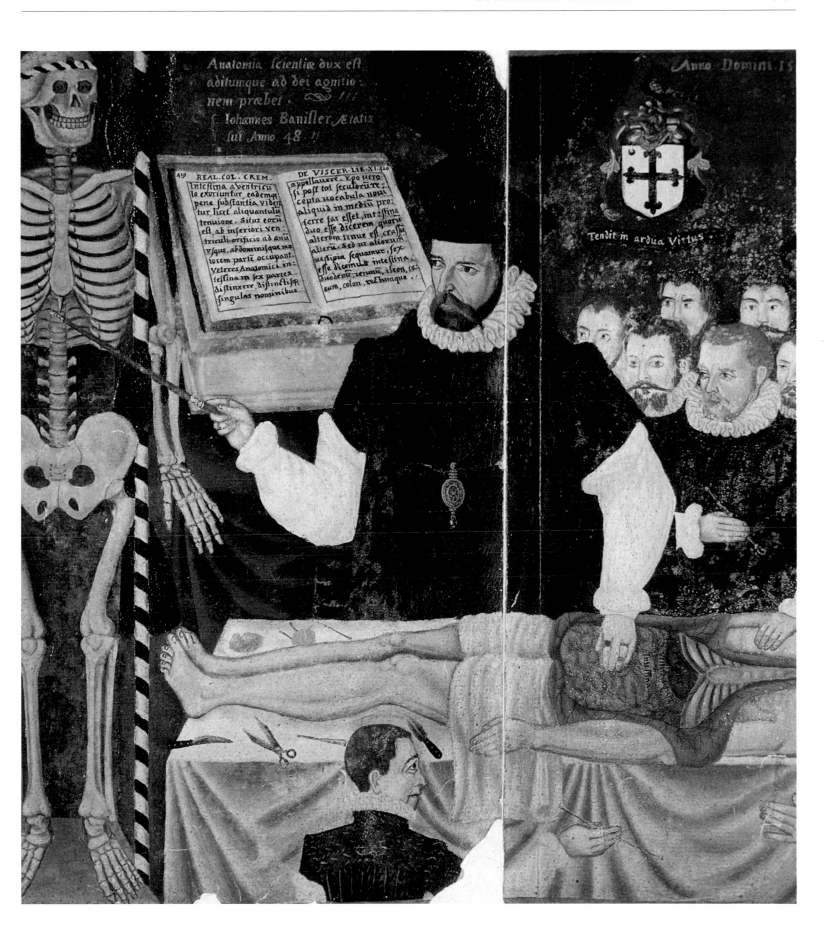

A strange and deadly malady swept parts of England in 1485, killing up to a third of the residents of the communities it visited. The disease reappeared in 1506, this time to halve the inhabitants of some towns and villages. A third eruption took place in 1517 and a fourth in 1528, when the illness was also said to be widespread in northern Europe. The pestilence appeared in England a final time in 1551 and then apparently vanished, leaving myriad unsolved puzzles in its wake.

This mysterious disease, dubbed 'sweating sickness', or *sudor anglicus*, and also known more simply as the 'English Sweat', or just plain 'Sweat', constitutes a great 'black hole' in historical epidemiology. Scholars who have agonized,

CHAPTER 24

SWEATING SICKNESS: AN ENGLISH MYSTERY

By Kenneth F. Kiple and Kriemhild Coneè Ornelas

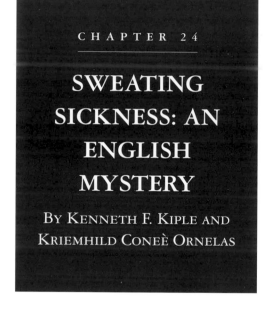

debated and speculated for centuries about the identity and origin of the ailment have made frustratingly little headway and many details, large and small, remain in dispute. The German epidemiologist August Hirsch wrote that the disease broke out in 1486 among troops, shortly after the battle of Bosworth Field, which brought the War of the Roses to a close. This battle for the throne of England was won by the army of the Duke of Richmond, Henry Tudor, who killed King Richard III and replaced him, as Henry VII.

Hirsch's translator, however, the British physician and medical historian Charles Creighton, wrote in his own work on the diseases of England that the initial outbreak occurred in London in 1485, arriving there with some of Henry's mercenaries just returned from France. The problem of whether to date this outbreak to 1486 or to 1485 (and all of the others until that of 1551) is due to the one-year discrepancy between the English and the Roman calendars. But the discrepancy as to the place of the initial appearance of the disease is not so easily resolved.

In the early sixteenth century the Italian Hieronymus Fracastorius, sometimes called the father of scientific epidemiology, thought that the Sweat was contagious, jumping from person to person and from town to town. By contrast, Hirsch stated emphatically that almost all contemporary observers had believed the disease not to be contagious and he made it clear that they had persuaded him.

Regardless of whether the sickness first appeared in London or among the soldiers at Bosworth Field it seems to have been the latter who, after disbanding, carried it all over England, though not into Scotland. In London the 'pestilence' or 'plague', as it was called, stunned the populace with a variety of dramatic lethal symptoms. It began without warning, generally at night or early morning. Chills and tremors were followed by high fever and great weakness. Perspiration covered the body and most observers reported a

rash. If the victim was to recover, the perspiration diminished to be replaced with an abundant flow of urine, and recovery was complete within a week, or two at the outside. In grave cases, by contrast, intense headache and convulsions were followed by coma, and death arrived with incredible speed. Many died a few hours after symptoms appeared although most lingered for twenty-four to forty-eight hours. Surviving the disease seems to have conferred no immunity and some, like Cardinal Wolsey, were said to have endured two or even three attacks in succession.

Unlike most epidemics, the Sweat, although not totally ignoring the poor, showed a preference for the better off – especially better-off males of middle age. Indeed the disease so humbled the important and the fashionable that the common people called it the 'stop-gallant'. During the first week of the epidemic in London it was reported to have permanently 'stopped' two Lord Mayors and six aldermen. At Oxford, panicked professors and students alike abandoned the university which was promptly shut down for six weeks. But in contrast with epidemics of other diseases this one, as a rule, spared children and the aged.

The malady inspired great fear in the population because of its incredibly swift course from onset to death. When it struck, economic activity ceased, and those who could flee, fled. However, compared with other epidemic diseases such as smallpox or plague, which tended to move steadily, and inexorably decimated the populations in their paths, the Sweat darted here and there, and although it could be devastating locally, probably had little or no overall demographic impact.

The first outbreak frustrated an impatient Henry by forcing postponement of his coronation. But five weeks after it struck the disease disappeared and Henry was crowned before the year was out. Perhaps he should have waited. Polydore Vergil, an Italian diplomat and scholar in London, wrote at the time that by appearing during the first year of Henry's reign, the Sweat was seen as a very bad omen.

The second eruption broke out in 1508, when King Henry VII was in the last months of his life. This time it

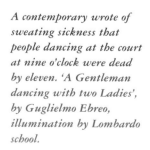

A contemporary wrote of sweating sickness that people dancing at the court at nine o'clock were dead by eleven. 'A Gentleman dancing with two Ladies', by Guglielmo Ebreo, illumination by Lombardo school.

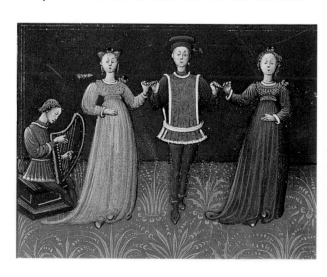

seems definitely to have begun in London and to have subsequently burst upon the faculties and students at both Oxford and Cambridge where it killed many distinguished scholars. Its stay, however, was apparently brief, and there is little record of it.

In 1517 Henry VIII was absorbed with weighing the advantages and disadvantages of playing balance-of-power politics with Spain and France. He was probably also alr scheming to have his name put forward as a candidate for Holy Roman Emperor when he was rudely torn away from these preoccupations by yet another appearance of the Sweat. The disease chased him and his court out of the capital and into refuge at Windsor. However, although Henry 'withdrew from all business on account of the pestilence' and had the good fortune to escape it, others around him were not so lucky. Indeed the King was doubtless apprehensive that his own luck was running out when the Sweat followed him to Windsor and killed many in his court.

Within six months the Sweat had spread over a great part of the countryside where it struck at random, killing from a third to one half of the populations in some of the hardest hit towns. Once again it brought death to many students and their teachers at Oxford and Cambridge, although as before it refrained from entering Scotland. A chronicler of the epidemic wrote that the malady sometimes killed its victims within three, even two hours and that a person merry at dinner could be dead by supper. Another wrote that people dancing at the court at nine o'clock were dead by eleven.

It is interesting to note how the disease seemed to spare the Irish (although something called a 'plague of sweating' appeared there in 1492), the Scots and the Welsh, but during this 1517 outbreak the pestilence was said to pursue Englishmen even on to the continent at Calais, where it singled out only Englishmen.

The first epidemic reputed to have affected people other than the English was the fourth, and perhaps most ferocious, eruption of the Sweat. This one – the outbreak of 1528 and 1529 – began as the others in London, spread rapidly across England and, as in the past, stopped at the Scottish border. Yet it reportedly did not stop short of the continent; rather, most believe that it engulfed it. According to Hirsch, the disease first appeared in Baltic and North Sea ports and from

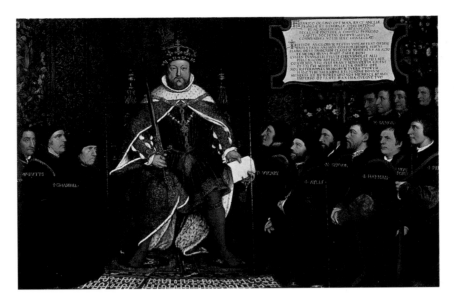

Henry VIII handing over a charter to Thomas Vicary, 1541, commemorating the joining of the Barbers and Surgeons guilds.

there extended over all of Germany, the Netherlands, Denmark, Sweden, Livonia, Lithuania, Russia, Poland and Switzerland. The Catholics of central Europe thought it God's retribution for Luther's heresies, basing their belief on the fact that France and the Catholic countries of southern Europe escaped completely.

At the time when the Sweat supposedly arrived, many in Germany were, however, already under siege by typhus and plague, while also contending with severe famine, making it impossible then or now to sort out the various illnesses. But there is no question that epidemic diseases, whatever they were, severely punished Germany. According to American physician and medical historian Hans Zinsser, at Göttingen mortality was such that five to eight corpses had to be placed in a single grave. In Marburg, disease interrupted the Council of the Reformation, and at Augsburg some 15,000 became ill in the first five days after an epidemic struck there.

Back in London, the Sweat continued to harass Henry VIII – this time by separating the ardent King from Anne Boleyn. It also terrorized the population to the point that social organization crumbled, agricultural activity ceased, and famine ensued.

Upon his death in 1547, Henry was succeeded by his son, Edward VI (1437–53), himself soon to die of 'consumption' (probably tuberculosis). The boy-king was on the throne when the Sweat of 1551 broke out, this time uncharacteristically not in London, but in Shrewsbury, where it was said to have killed 900 people in just a few days. Characteristically, however, it halted at the Scottish border after overrunning England. Rumors circulated that the

Engraving of Johannes Caius, by C. Ammon Junior, 1650. Caius wrote a book on how to survive sweating sickness, which appeared a year after the disease vanished.

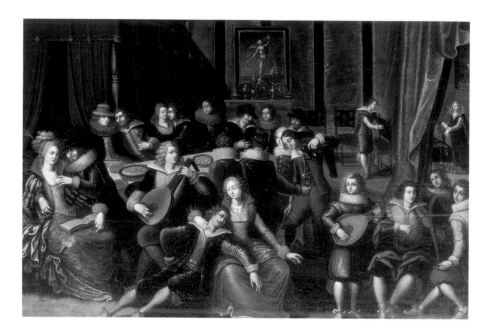

'Scène Galante in a Château' by Louis de Caullery (c. 1580– 1621). Known by the common people as 'stop-gallant', the disease was believed by some to have originated in France.

disease was once again afflicting the English abroad; it was also said that foreigners in England were exempt from its ravages.

In dealing with the English sweating sickness the easy part is sketching out the epidemics. The hard part – its identification – has yet to be accomplished with certainty by anyone. A major difficulty is the incredibly savage sea of pestilence that was continually washing over England at that time. In the sixteenth century bubonic plague, smallpox and measles all coexisted at various places and times to hammer populations. Outbreaks of typhus were frequent; influenza periodically reached the island from the continent; and there was plenty of malignant syphilis about. It is because of this pottage of pathogens that some who have pondered the question of the identity of the Sweat have tended to view it as a somewhat different manifestation of one of these all-too-familiar epidemic ailments.

For example, because of the spots or rash occasioned by sweating sickness, a finger has been pointed at typhus as a likely candidate. But Zinsser, who probably knew more about typhus than anyone else, discounted this explanation because of the lightning-fast onset of the Sweat and the speed with which it caused death.

On the other hand, the rapid onset as well as the haphazard manner of spread, seemed to focus suspicion on influenza – a disease well known for its instability and unnerving ability to mutate quickly from a relatively mild illness to a lethal one. But the apparent absence of any respiratory symptoms or secondary cases of pneumonia loom as prominent exonerating factors; nonetheless, according to some, influenza remains high on the list of suspects.

Others have viewed the sweating sickness as some sort of streptococcal infection like acute rheumatic fever, but such a theory has attracted few adherents. Meningitis, which can develop into a fulminating blood infection, might be another

possibility. When this occurs, sudden prostration, high fever and skin blotches are common and death can occur within hours. But an eliminating factor is that even in epidemics of meningitis, relatively few individuals in the populations at risk develop any symptoms of clinical disease at all.

The sixteenth-century physician Johannes Caius, who attended three Tudor sovereigns (Edward VI, Mary and Elizabeth) and was elected president of the Royal College of Physicians in 1555, wrote a guide for the public on how to avoid or, failing that, survive the English 'Sweatyng Sickness'. In his *Boke against the Sweate*, written in 1522, Caius took note of the special susceptibility of the English and blamed it on beer in particular and their diet in general. But because the book was written in the year after the final outbreak of the pestilence, Caius's theories were not put to the test. It was only later that scholars built on Caius's diet theory, noting that, since the Sweat seemed partial to the better-off, the problem might have been caused by access to some of the more expensive foods, one or more of which had triggered a kind of food poisoning that, like ergotism, could bring on circulatory collapse.

But circulatory collapse can also be produced by severe dehydration, such as that seen so often in the nineteenth century among cholera patients; and in that century of cholera pandemics physicians routinely purged patients already suffering severely from dehydration which meant they were cooperating with the disease in killing its victims. It has been speculated that such a partnership between illness and physician may also have been established during the Sweat epidemics, which would presumably explain why the financially better-off suffered disproportionately compared to the rest of the population: as a group, they were among those most able to afford the doctors.

Creighton, however, writing in 1891, blamed the French. He believed that the disease was harbored and nurtured in the soils of the lower basin of the Seine; that it had initially been brought from France to England by the Flemish mercenaries of Henry VII; that weather conditions had subsequently been responsible for its return; and that the French had lived with the Sweat long enough to have acquired some immunity against it – something which was not true of his own countrymen.

Creighton's epidemiological point about the extreme susceptibility of the English is an important one, even if one is not prepared to concede the possibility that the disease somehow blew capriciously across the English Channel from time to time. Zinsser also speculated that the Sweat had come from the continent – in the form of a virus. Like Creighton, he believed that the illness existed there in a mild form because its people had a long history of exposure to it and, consequently, had developed a relative immunity to it. But because the English had enjoyed no such long-standing intimacy with the virus, they proved almost totally susceptible whenever they had contact with it.

Such a theory would explain why foreigners in England were reputed to escape the Sweat, while the English remained

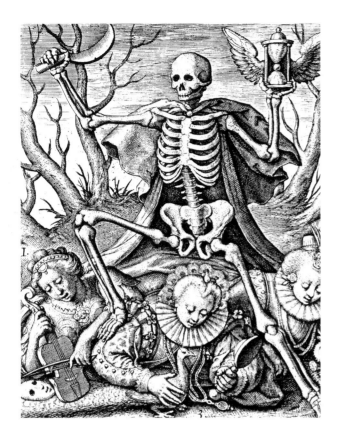

susceptible abroad. It might even account for the mysterious disappearance of the disease, which may not have disappeared at all, but have simply become quietly endemic in England in a mild form after the five epidemics had weeded out the most susceptible and educated the immune systems of the remainder.

The difficulty with this explanation, satisfying as it is, is that it sheds no light on the apparent total exemption of Scotland to the Sweat, and an at least partial exemption of Ireland and Wales. This brings us to another very intriguing hypothesis put forth on the origin of the Sweat which suggests that it was actually the result of some arbovirus transmitted by an insect vector – like the yellow fever virus which is vectored by various mosquito species. Some support for this argument is provided by Hirsch who unearthed the information that the appearance of sweating sickness was invariably preceded by heavy rains and, in some places, considerable flooding – both of which would have dramatically encouraged mosquito proliferation. Moreover, with a little dexterity in ecological research, this theory might account for the absence of the disease in Scotland and, perhaps, Wales because of the mountainous (and thus colder) terrain, and in Ireland because of the protection provided by another channel to leap.

Many unanswered questions remain about the vector; even more so in the matter of the origin of the arbovirus. For one thing, arboviruses are generally tropical residents and England is hardly tropical. It is true, however, that the Portuguese had been in close touch with Africa – the home

of so many arboviruses – on the one hand, and England on the other, almost since Philippa of Lancaster married Joâo I and their famous son Henry the Navigator began launching expeditions down the African coast in the fifteenth century. But in an era when ships were ponderous and slow, the odds of carrying such a virus even once from the coast of Africa to Lisbon, and then transshipping it northward to England, seem improbable. For it to have happened five times seems impossible.

Such tortuous speculations make a broader canvas increasingly appealing – a larger historical picture which reminds us that, although the Sweat may seem singular, sweating sicknesses are not. Ancients like Celsus and Galen described diseases that had similar symptoms, and Hirsch, among others, was intrigued with the identity of the Picardy sweat (or miliary fever) of France and its possible relationship to the English sweating sickness. He wrote that the first 'unambiguous' outbreak he could identify took place in 1718, and until the end of the eighteenth century the illness had been limited to the north and east of France. By the nineteenth century, however, it had become one of the most widely diffused diseases in the country. Hirsch counted 194 epidemics between 1718 and 1879, with most limited to a single village or a few localities.

He noted that in addition to limited diffusion, outbreaks of the Picardy Sweat were similar to the English Sweat in that they were of very short duration, began explosively, and its victims displayed many of the same symptoms as the English sufferers. On the other hand, although Hirsch is somewhat contradictory regarding its lethal nature, it would seem that unlike the Sweat, this disease, as a rule, caused few deaths. Nonetheless he claimed to have no doubt of a close similarity between the two. However, he also found a close similarity between miliary fever and cholera, and save for dehydration, none of those seized by the Sweat in England were said to have cholera-like symptoms.

We have solved no mystery here, merely examined its contours. The Sweat remains a biological artifact of its own time and serves as a reminder of how pathogenically perilous those days actually were and how incredibly fatalistic those who lived through them must have been.

BIBLIOGRAPHY

Carmichael, Ann G. 1993. 'Sweating Sickness', in Kenneth F. Kiple (ed.), *The Cambridge World History of Human Disease*. Cambridge, England and New York.

Hecker, J. F. K. 1844. *Epidemics of the Middle Ages* (trans. B. G. Babbington). London.

Hirsch, August. 1883–6. *Handbook of Historical and Geographical Pathology* (trans. Charles Creighton), 3 vols. London.

McGrew, Roderick E. 1985. *Encyclopedia of Medical History*. New York.

Shrewsbury, J. F. D. 1970. *A History of Bubonic Plague in the British Isles.* Cambridge, England.

Wylie, John A. H. and Leslie H. Collier. 1981. 'The English Sweating Sickness (Sudor Anglicus): A Reappraisal', *Journal of the History of Medicine and Allied Sciences*, 36, pp. 425–45.

An engraving by Hieronymus Wierx giving a graphic interpretation of death laying low the ladies of the Elizabethan court.

Chlorosis is a most peculiar disease. It had its heyday in the late nineteenth century, when all adolescent girls seen by European and American physicians seemed to have at least a 'touch' of it, yet by the third decade of the twentieth century, it had become rare. Physicians diagnosed chlorosis, or the 'green sickness', in teenage girls who were pale, weak, tired and nervous, who suffered from palpitations, breathlessness, indigestion, constipation, irregular menstrual periods and odd appetites. What is this disease, that ran so rampant in the last century and disappeared in this one?

Many historians have addressed the issue. One of the first problems to be settled is the name, which means literally 'a state of greenness'. Were chlorotic girls green? 'It would take the eye of faith to see any justification for the title of the disease,' an American physician who had seen hundreds of cases commented in 1915. 'If one exercises a great deal of imagination, one may possibly see the slightest imaginable tint of olive green in the shadow beneath the chin, but that is all. To the ordinary eye, the color is a yellowish pallor in brunettes and a whitish, although extreme, pallor in blondes.' In the words of an historian, 'the green skin color of chlorosis … remains, like the origin of syphilis, one of the more fascinating problems in the history of disease'. One researcher, perhaps facetiously, suggested that the green color arose from compression of the gall bladder and liver by corseting, disrupting bilirubin metabolism. A thorough review of publications on chlorosis found that out of nineteen descriptive papers on the disease, only three made any mention of the greenish hue of the patients. It seems probable that chlorotic patients, on the whole, were not green at all.

It is more likely that the greenness in question did not refer to skin color, which seems to have been more pale pink or gray, but was an allusion to the age and immaturity of the patients. Shakespeare used the term in that sense, when he had Juliet's father rage at her for not agreeing to his marriage plans:

'mistress minion, you
Thank me no thankings, nor proud me no prouds,
But fettle your fine joints 'gainst Thursday next,
To go with Paris to St Peter's church,
Or I will drag thee on a hurdle thither.
Out, you green sickness carrion! Out, you baggage!'
(*Romeo and Juliet*, Act III)

Nineteenth-century physicians would occasionally report a yellow-green tinge to their chlorotics' skin, but most mentioned instead their paleness. Almost all, however,

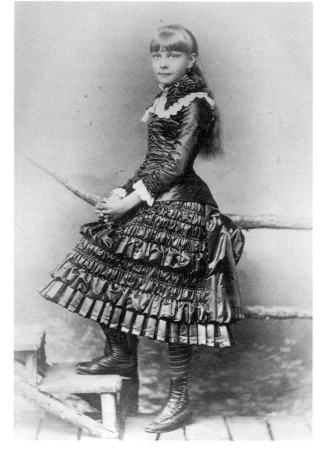

limited this diagnosis to females under twenty-five, exactly those who are the most 'green' in the sense of immature.

The earliest mention of the illness is suggested in certain fragmentary Hippocratic writings, but appears definitively in a 1554 account on the *morbus virgineus* (virgin's sickness) by Johannes Lange. This physician described the afflictions of one Anna, whose father is unable to marry her off because of her ill health. The list of symptoms resembles that of nineteenth-century chlorosis: 'Her face which last year showed rosy cheeks and lips, has become pale and bloodless, her heart palpitates at every movement … she loses her breath when dancing or going upstairs, she dislikes her food, especially meat, and her legs swell toward the evening.' Lange believed the diagnosis was obvious – the lady was suffering from 'love fever'. What she needed was marriage, followed by the fulfillment of sexual intercourse and motherhood.

Paleness was the lover's badge after all, as Ovid said: 'Paleat omnis amans, hic est color aptus amanti.' Pining, weeping and faintness was to be expected from a girl whose mind and body were first awakening to love. Jean Varandal coined the term 'chlorosis' for this love ailment in 1620, and again recommended marriage and motherhood as a treatment. Other terms also reflected the association with adolescent, innocent girls, such as *pallor virginium*, *foedi virginium colores*, *febris virginia* and *cachexia virgineum*. While physicians referred to it frequently in the seventeenth and

Could chlorosis have been caused by corsets, and the subsequent compression of the gall-bladder? Young girls were the primary sufferers.

eighteenth centuries, it was only in the nineteenth that chlorosis became an epidemic among white girls of England, France and the United States.

Chlorosis was a disease of city girls, and so carried a certain aura of refinement. Isaac Walton in his *The Compleat Angler* tells the sad tale of a man who wed such a delicate woman:

'I married a wife of late,
The more's my unhappy fate:
I married her for love
As my fancy did me move,
And not for a worldly estate:
But oh! The green-sickness
Soon changed her likeness;
And all her beauty did fail
But 'tis not so
Wirh those that go
Thro' frost and snow
As all men know
And carry the milking-pail.'

In other words, rural girls did not get chlorosis, whatever it was. But poor girls certainly could. The disease was also seen commonly in female factory workers under the age of twenty-five, whose weakness and other symptoms would land them in charity hospitals. In 1923, for example, Dr J. M. H. Campbell published his study of 130 cases of chlorosis at Guy's Hospital, and compared them to several thousand others documented at other hospitals in London, Sheffield, Birmingham and Glasgow. His patients were working girls, living in crowded, airless tenements.

So this was a city disease, afflicting adolescent girls of both straitened and affluent circumstances, who lived in urban areas, which peaked in the last two decades of the nineteenth century. Multiple explanations were offered for the cause of the illness. Bad air was central to many – the closed stale air of the drawing room or the dust-filled atmosphere of the factory. This was accompanied by a lack of exercise in the fresh air, either due to indolence among the fashionable or the restrictions of poverty and work among the poor. In an era when foul odors arising as miasms from swamps and decaying animal matter were widely blamed for a panoply of diseases, the possibility that bad air could be toxic was easily believed, and the invigorating, tonic effect of fresh air hailed by all physicians.

Dress was just as frequently blamed. This was the age of the corset and the hoop skirt, which significantly limited movement. Not for these girls the loose flowing dresses of Jane Austen's heroines, who are frequently found strolling in the garden or galloping over the fields, and who never worry about their waistlines. Rather this is the world of Scarlet O'Hara, who is enjoined by her maid to 'eat like a bird' if she would lead her beau to the altar, and is laced so tightly that her waist shrinks to eighteen inches. It was an era when the beautiful girl was languorous and pale, with just a hint of consumption. It was also an era when more and more young women were working in factories. These factors combined to help create chlorosis.

Some physicians targeted puberty itself as the danger. Nineteenth-century medical thought tended to see the uterus as the central organ in a woman's body, and one from which many derangements flowed. It was, as one American physician explained in the 1870s, 'as if the Almighty, in creating the female sex, had taken the uterus and built up a woman around it'. Girls were frail, irritable and prone to nervous diseases – particularly during puberty, when the uterus awakened to its central function. All of a girl's energies were needed to emerge safely from this turbulent period. Physicians worried that if teenage girls devoted too much attention to mental work and study, it would threaten their health. The 'nervous force' thus wasted on books was required for the healthy onset of menstruation and growth into normal womanhood. Such a misspent youth could lead to chlorosis, or else the state of nervous exhaustion called neurasthenia. Girls would do better to behave more like children – eat abundantly, run and play outdoors in loose-fitting clothing – rather than cramping their bodies in fashionable dress, often

Line engraving of Johannes Lange by T. de Bry, 1645. Lange was a famous Renaissance physician, who first described chlorosis.

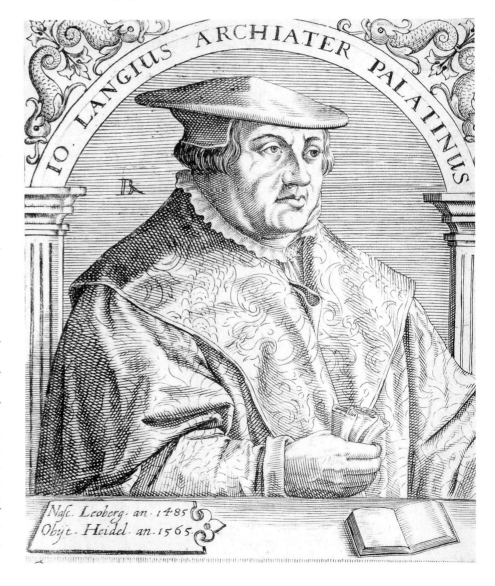

IO LANGIUS ARCHIATER PALATINUS

Nasc. Leoberg. an. 1485
Obijt. Heidel. an. 1565

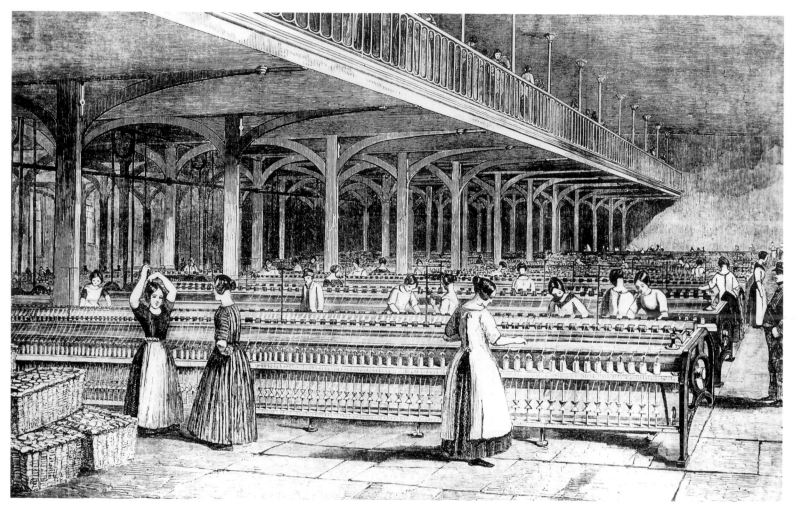

Chlorosis was essentially a city disease, commonly found in young female factory workers. The dust-filled atmosphere and bad air was believed to be a causal factor of the illness.

with the breasts dangerously exposed, and limiting their activities to reading and needlepoint.

From the mid nineteenth century onward physicians began to seek more precise understanding of the organic site of chlorosis. The German physician and pathologist Rudolf Virchow thought he found it in congenital abnormalities of the heart and blood vessels. Another physician targeted a specific malfunction of the uterus and ovaries, leading to the release of toxins throughout the body. A third believed that the internal rearrangement of the digestive organs caused by tight lacing was itself the source of chlorosis. A fourth argued that constipation led to an autointoxication when the body absorbed poisons from the retained feces. Still another held that chlorosis was a nervous disorder which resulted from the evils of masturbation. None of these theories explained more than a fraction of the cases, however, and a better answer was needed.

The theory most commonly put forward from the mid nineteenth century onward was that chlorosis was a form of anemia. With increasing refinements in technology physicians were able to quantify the deficiency of red blood cells, the oxygen-carrying compound called hemoglobin, and the presence of elemental iron in the bodies of chlorotic girls.

Physicians then, and some historians in retrospect, announced that chlorosis was iron-deficiency anemia, and the mystery was solved.

There is abundant evidence for this view. The diet of chlorotic girls might well have been short on iron-rich meat, eggs and green vegetables. either due to poverty or personal preference. Eating meat was associated with crude passionate male behavior; girls ate more delicate foods. Adolescent girls require extra iron during their growth spurts, just when the onset of menstruation robs them of this valuable resource. The disease's symptoms are also consistent with anemia. Anemic patients are weak, tired and short of breath, since without enough iron the blood does a poor job of carrying oxygen throughout the body. The heart beats more rapidly in an attempt to make up for this deficit by pushing the iron-poor blood through more often. A pale complexion results, since it is iron that gives the red blood cell its color. Those who argued that chlorosis was merely an early term for iron-deficiency anemia pointed to the universal success of iron tonics in treating the disease.

Iron deficiency can result from two separate processes. One is inadequate intake in foods, and the other is excessive loss from the body. Women lose iron in menstrual blood, and during pregnancy. But there are other causes of blood loss. One is therapeutic bloodletting, the creation of anemia by the doctor's lancet. The other is the loss of blood from the gastrointestinal tract, such as from ulcers, a frequent problem among chlorotic patients. Yet iron deficiency anemia should have been equally or more common among older persons, especially women who had borne several children, lived on a diet scanty in meat, and suffered from the heavy menstrual bleeding common to women in their forties. The iron deficiency hypothesis explains much, but not why teenage girls were specifically affected.

One curious symptom exhibited by chlorotic girls supports the anemia hypothesis. They had very strange food preferences, characterized by (according to one 1875 source): 'loss of appetite, loathing of food, and often a desire which almost amounts to a passion, for such indigestible and repulsive articles as charcoal, slate-stones, chalk, plaster, flies, bugs, and other similar substances'. Another author mentioned they would only eat the more charred portions of meat. This behavior is called pica. It has mostly been associated with hookworm disease, a parasitic infestation that causes severe iron-deficiency anemia, which was once prevalent in Italy and the American South, and still occurs in parts of Africa. Pregnant women and children will also eat clay and other odd items. No one knows what leads anemic people to chew on such things, but the therapeutic use of iron usually ends this tendency.

This behavior may lead to another explanation for chlorosis, however. In their loathing for food, and ingestion of such substances as vinegar to make them slimmer, the chlorotic girls resemble modern anorexia nervosa sufferers. This disease coincides with the age and gender range of chlorosis much better than does iron-deficiency anemia, which if anything should be more pronounced in women in their thirties and forties. I. S. L. Loudon has been one of the proponents of this view, that chlorosis was a manifestation of a 'psychological reaction to the turbulence of puberty and adolescence'. Some feminist historians have seen chlorosis as a disease of feminine resistance, a way to fend off womanhood, or, on the other hand, a way to grow to adulthood by mimicking the behavior of their frequently ill and invalid mothers. These viewpoints all share the assumption that chlorosis was some sort of mental

phenomenon or disorder, and that the remainder of the symptoms were secondary to this mental illness.

Anorexia nervosa, as a synonym for chlorosis, would account for another of its symptoms: irregular menstrual function. Though healthy teenage girls can suffer from it, the tendency to menstrual irregularity is heightened if the body becomes too thin, and the production of estrogen drops. Researchers have posited that this is a natural protective reflex of the body in response to famine conditions. If the woman does not menstruate, her uterus is not hospitable to a fertilized egg, and she will not get pregnant. In the teenager, the development of her secondary sexual characteristics will stop as well, so her chest will remain flat, pubic hair will be scanty, and the fat deposits that make for a curvaceous adult female will be delayed. It has often been put forward as one reason why anorexic girls persist in their self-starvation that they are either deliberately or subconsciously postponing maturity and the psychic stresses of sexual development. Of course, lacking sufficient nourishment, they are pale and weak. That factory

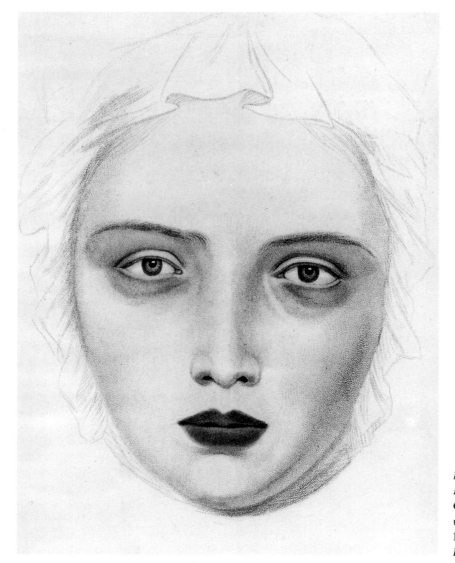

Plate depicting chlorosis in Marshall Hall, Commentaries on some of the more important of the Diseases of Females, *London, 1827.*

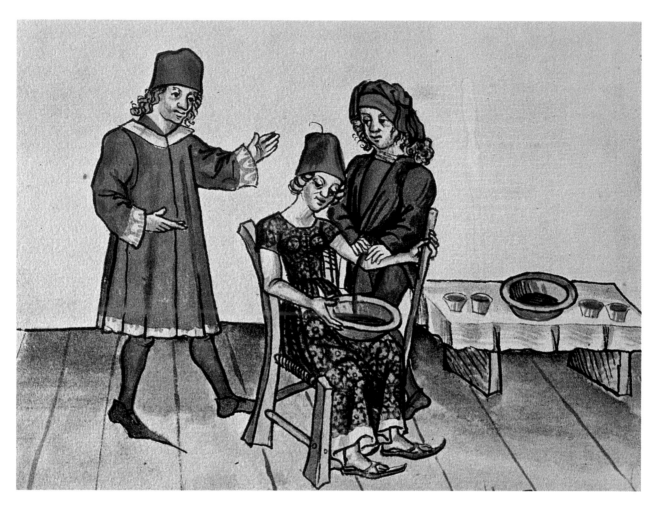

Blood-letting in Germany. Chlorotic girls could have been suffering from anaemia.

girls who suffered from malnutrition were lumped with these affluent girls into one diagnosis also makes sense in this light.

The list of chlorosis symptoms is so non-specific that it opens the door to a broad range of diagnoses. It is likely that chlorotic girls included those with iron-deficiency anemia, anorexia nervosa and a host of other illness. Certainly many of these pale, weak, breathless girls had tuberculosis, especially those working in dusty factories and living in crowded, poorly ventilated tenements. Some probably suffered from the available medications that were taken as tonics, including the popular 'Fowler's Solution', which contained arsenic and produced a pale complexion, as well as chronic arsenic poisoning. Others sipped laudanum, a tincture of opium, to alleviate pains and boredom. It is probable that there was a certain amount of hypochondria, in an effort to obtain attention. Scattered among these cases were girls with thyroid disease, renal failure, peptic ulcer disease, mitral valve stenosis (critical narrowing of a heart valve) and adrenal insufficiency. The last of these, known as Addison's disease, was more common then than now, for it could be a manifestation of tuberculosis. All told, it is foolish to try to determine that chlorosis was any one disorder, and more appropriate to conclude that physicians used the term for a variety of adolescent female illnesses.

One thing that is clear is that the disease disappeared early in the twentieth century. A physician who published 'Chlorosis – an Obituary' in 1936 asked, 'What disease, however, can compare with chlorosis in having occupied such a prominent place in medical practice only to disappear spontaneously while we are still speculating as to its etiology?' Although historians have not been able to answer this query conclusively, there have been some pertinent suggestions. One is improving diagnostic skill. With the chest X-ray becoming common in the second decade of the twentieth century, tuberculosis would have been harder to miss. The increasing frequency of chemical urinalysis would have cut out those with failing kidneys from the general diagnosis of chlorosis. This period also saw greater sophistication in diagnosing thyroid and other endocrine abnormalities. And an increased emphasis on the routine blood count made anemia a more familiar diagnostic category for physicians. The label chlorosis was shattered into the condition's constituent parts.

But that seems unlikely to be the full answer, especially for a disease that some said could be diagnosed at a glance. There are many reasons why physicians were apparently not seeing as many pale, breathless, weak teenage girls. The early twentieth-century girl was more active, with physical education classes common in schools and the corset on its way out. No longer was the beautiful girl a waif lingering on the edge of fainting, but rather the sturdy Gibson girl ready for a round of tennis. Maintaining such energy required a healthy appetite, and eating meat became fashionable again. Women were riding bicycles, climbing mountains and marching to secure the vote. For the factory workers, tuberculosis was on the decline and living conditions had improved. Greater regulation of the patent medicine industry reduced the use of arsenic compounds for the complexion, and laudanum use declined.

Of course something like chlorosis survives in all doctor's consulting rooms today. Now the girls are diagnosed with depression or panic disorder or even chronic fatigue syndrome, after the organic problems of anemia, thyroid dysfunction or renal disease have been ruled out by a few simple blood tests; and anorexia nervosa is still a major problem. But it is likely that the peculiar combination of factors that created the epidemic of chlorosis among nineteenth-century teenage girls, no longer exists.

BIBLIOGRAPHY
Brumberg, Joan. 1982. 'Chlorotic Girls, 1870–1920: A Historical Perspective on Female Adolescence', *Child Development* 53, pp. 1468–77.
Campbell, J. M. H. 1923. 'Chlorosis: A Study of the Guy's Hospital Cases During the Last Thirty Years, With Some Remarks on Its Etiology and the Causes of Its Diminished Frequency', *Guy's Hospital Reports* 73, pp. 247–97.
Figlio, Karl. 1978. 'Chlorosis and Chronic Disease in Nineteenth-Century Britain: The Social Constitution of Somatic Illness in a Capitalist Society', *Social History* 3, pp. 167–97.
Fowler, W. M. 1936. 'Chlorosis – An Obituary', *Annals of Medical History* 8, pp. 168–77.
Hudson, Robert P. 1977. 'The Biography of Disease: Lessons from Chlorosis', *Bulletin of the History of Medicine* 51, pp. 448–58.
Loudon, I. S. L. 1980. 'Chlorosis, Anaemia, and Anorexia Nervosa', *British Medical Journal* 281, pp. 1669–75.
Siddall, A. Clair. 1982. 'Chlorosis – Etiology Reconsidered', *Bulletin of the History of Medicine* 56, pp. 254–60.
Theriot, Nancy M. 1996. *Mothers and Daughters in Nineteenth-Century America: The Biosocial Construction of Femininity.* Lexington, Kentucky.

'Young Woman on her Death Bed', by Flemish schoo, seventeenth century.

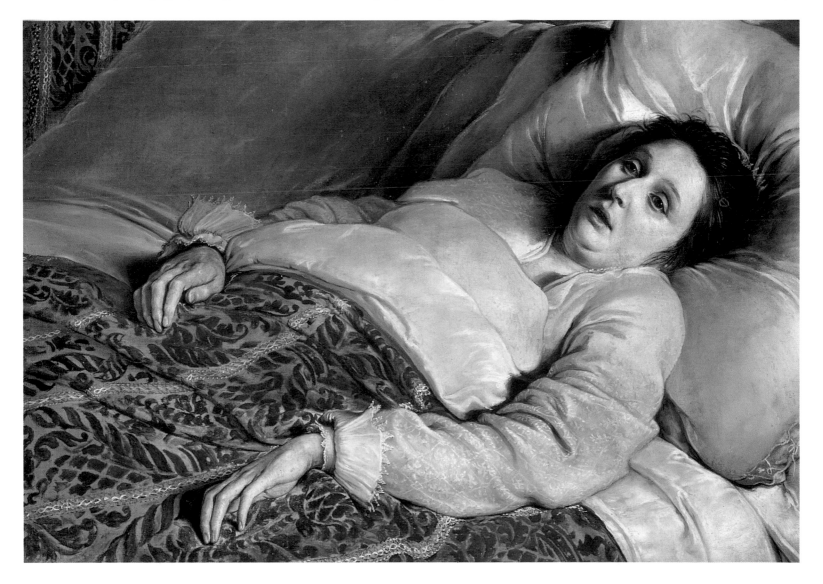

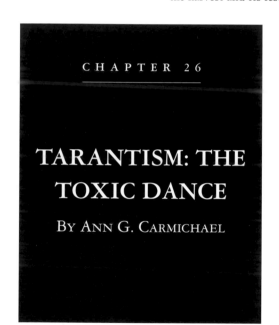

CHAPTER 26

TARANTISM: THE TOXIC DANCE

By Ann G. Carmichael

What is tarantism? What kind of disease is or was it? Indeed, what understanding of the terms 'disease' and 'epidemic' apply? Tarantism's history tells us far more about the history of our changing ideas and definitions of disease than about empirical realities.

Above all tarantism fits the standard modern definition of an epidemic – a clustering of illness events in space and time – for the phenomenon was quite localized to Apulia in the seventeenth and eighteenth centuries. In summer in southeast Italy the terrain is a scorched and impoverished; spiders, lizards, snakes and mad dogs emerge from the dusty earth and steal into the huts of poor farmers. In this parched landscape, just before the harvest and its festivals, emerge the strange sounds and sights of the *tarantati*. The victims are bitten by a tarantula – often being unable to recall when; frequently even the physical evidence of a bite is difficult to prove. The 'patient' declines, anorectic and listless, until the sounds of the traditional music produces both the diagnosis and the cure. If the cause of illness were truly from the tarantula, the *tarantato* or *tarantata* would respond by dancing, at first with a slow, snaky writhing, eventually with an accelerated, flailing motion, until exhausted. Frequently the musicians could not keep up, needing to break long before the dance was through, but if they did not outlast the victim's dance, the bite of the tarantula might continue to effect its power in years to come.

In an attempt to get at the 'facts' of tarantism, a physician practicing in Lecce, Epifanio Ferdinando, in his *Hundred Medical Histories or Observations* of 1621, told the tale of a boy named Pietro Simone di Messapia, bitten in the night, and seized with pain. He couldn't stand up; he felt he was suffocating; he sweated profusely. But he was fully recovered within the week, thanks to the dance. Ferdinando then launched an inquiry into the nature of the tarantula, and assumed that he was seeking a particular variety of poisonous spider. He also had a second objective, of considerable interest to his contemporaries: the possibility of the cure of a disease through music. Ferdinando compiled a list of specific questions to guide the investigation of other cases. For example, was dancing necessary to cure the symptoms? How did patients respond to theriac, a popular antidote to many poisons?

Ferdinando was well aware that many scholars questioned the reality of the disease and its cure. Already the scientific and medical community wanted to distinguish the true *tarantati* from the phonies, as well as the true methods of healing from the actions of charlatans and other cunning men. True *tarantati* were bitten by a tarantula, and were cured by dancing to a tarantella.

The dance known as the Tarantella was socalled because it mimicked the behaviour of those afflicted by tarantism.

Ferdinando's younger contemporary, the Jesuit father Athanasius Kircher (1602-80), also collected case reports from Apulia. Kircher, who had no medical training, was far more interested in understanding how music might heal and what effects it had upon the humors, than in the cause of the phenomenon. As a scriptor at the Collegio Romano, Kircher might have taken a moral interest in exposing the lascivious undercurrents of a quasi-pagan ritual among superstitious people, but instead, typical of polymaths, he was sidetracked into an ever-deepening interest in the music that cured (the tarantella), its instruments, precise tempos and harmonic clauses. He described pipes, flutes, various kinds of drums, harps, zithers and timbrels, among others. He recorded the affinity that victims felt with certain colors, the need to be surrounded by an array of ribbons, the decidedly amorous gestures embedded in the dance. These were banalities unworthy of serious study, but Kircher was notoriously gullible, even to the point of believing in flying dragons.

Giorgio Baglivi, who was well known in the late seventeenth century for his newer 'modern' understanding of physics and mechanics within medical theory, was adopted and raised by an Apulian physician, and he rekindled interest in the problem of tarantism, borrowing from his adopted father's first-hand case observations. The afflicted sometimes danced wildly, demanding bright colors, reacting especially violently to the color black. Others tore their clothes, almost to nudity, waving ribbons or red cloths as they danced. Some howled; other clawed holes in the baked

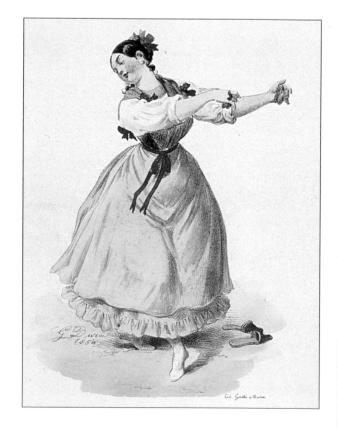

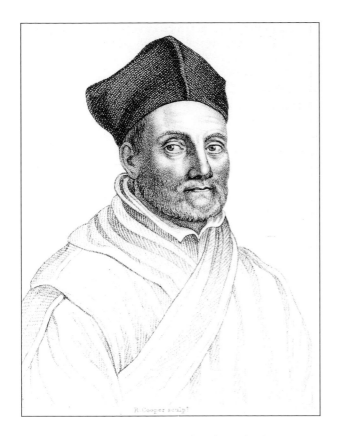

earth. The music meanwhile played 'with the greatest quickness imaginable'.

Baglivi's treatise was published only in 1738, by which time a firmer taxonomy of basic animal and insect species existed. The tarantula, as had been noted for over a century, was widespread in Europe and nowhere else was it poisonous. Baglivi assumed, as others had, that the Apulian species was unique. He captured a spider, procured its bite on the lip of a rabbit and carefully detailed the animal's five-day illness: difficulty in breathing, refusal of food and drink, ultimately overcome by coma. He summoned musicians, but the rabbit did not dance and was not cured – calling into question regional reports of bitten wasps and chickens, even the tarantula itself, being healed by the tarantella.

Baglivi divided the *tarantati* into the false and the true, the latter suffering genuine poisoning through a spider's bite. Music, he declared, was ineffective or unnecessary in true cases – a reversal in the logic that confounds the very definition of tarantism. He found that the false cases were responsive to music, and that they were almost exclusively young women. Thus false tarantism became a cultural-psychic phenomenon, which could be related to witchcraft and hysteria. Baglivi noted that many skeptics called tarantism *Il carnevaletto delle donne* – the little Mardi Gras (or Carnival) for women.

Moving on from the Scientific Revolution to the Enlightenment, we come to Francesco Serao (1702–83), who produced three ponderous tomes devoted to proving tarantism a popular superstition. The force of the belief, he argued, propelled unfortunate peasants into a profound melancholy, risking death if they were not aroused with music. Serao, secretary of the Academy of Sciences for the realm of Naples, provided an exacting classification and anatomical discussion of the spider, finding no evidence for a toxin, despite Baglivi's claim. Next he moved to an historical survey, beginning with the fifteenth and sixteenth centuries. Wondering why the music seemed to cure some people, Serao hypothesized that the toxicity of the tarantula was not comparable to well-known reptilian, insect and animal poisons. Instead it was a 'psychic' toxin, inducing melancholy.

At this point we skip ahead 200 years, to the decades following World War II. Possibly through the extensive involvement of southern Italy as a theater of combat and the postwar government's attempts to redress the extreme economic differences between the rural south and the industrial north, scholars once again became involved in the problem of tarantism. Postwar Apulia attracted Ernesto De Martino, an influential historian of religion and folklore. Cases of tarantism still occurred there and De Martino assembled a team of investigators, including physicians, to observe and record new cases. He was conscious both that many folkloric studies were taken out of their full historical and social context, and that tarantism as a medical phenomenon raised issues of what was a 'real' disease. The expedition to the wilds of Apulia took place in 1959, and De Martino published his findings in 1961, in *La terra del rimorso*, or 'Land of Remorse', a study of religion in the south focusing on the symbolic systems involved in healing.

De Martino paid renewed attention to the effects of the Apulian tarantula's bite. It is not lethal, but does cause swelling and inflammation of the area bitten, also edema, nausea and vomiting, vertigo and agitation. The exaggerated reaction of the Pugliese to the bite thus occupied a 'gray zone' between pharmacology and psychiatry. However his attention was fixed most on the gestures, signs and words associated with announcement of affliction. The victim was typically female and had sensed that a bite had occurred at some point in the past. A lapse of time between the bite and the illness was usual, but even years could go by. Typically, the victim was bitten in her youth, and the report of illness came in midsummer, close to the annual festival of Saints Peter and Paul.

De Martino argued that control of the dancing was the key to resolving both the illness and the disturbance it imposed on the community. Often the first scene of the dance was domestic, with neighbors milling about, bringing sheets and ribbons to

The Jesuit A. Kircher (1602–80) had no medical training, and was far more interested in how music might affect the humors.

Giorgio Baglivi (1669–1707) published a treatise on tarantism declaring music to be ineffective in true cases.

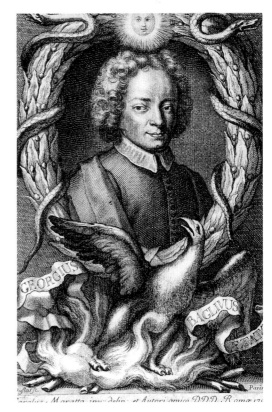

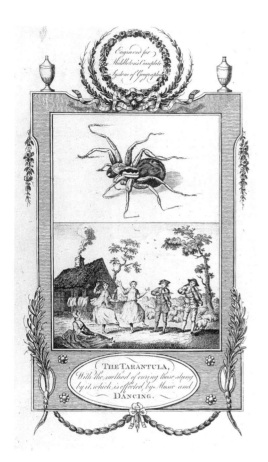

'Engraved for Middleton's Complete System of Geography. The Tarantula. With the method of curing those stung by it which is effected by music and dancing.'

'The Dancing Mania.' Engraving (1642) after Pieter Breughel.

aid in the cure. A space was created, inside or out, delineating boundaries for the ever-quickening dance. Ribbons of many colors were thrown on the sheet or ceremonial perimeter. An older man had to make the diagnosis, and an older woman, a person of some authority in the community, directed the assemblage of musicians, even set the rhythms by playing the tambourine. As in Kircher's day, a musical cure proved the cause.

In the 1950s, a second phase of the drama was also important. *Tarentati* who were not quickly cured had to be taken to the church of San Paolo a Galatina, in Lecce. (This is the town where Ferdinando Kircher's informants and Baglivi's father had worked.) There the effect of the poison could be exorcised with the aid of holy water or relics. Jervis, a member of the research team assembled by De Martino, took extensive personal histories of the afflicted and decided that the victims were 'acting out' individual sufferings and frustrations, that the dance represented, in psychiatric terms, a dissociative episode or psychotic break. He found a few mistaken diagnoses – one otitis media, or severe inner ear infection, and a few instances of epilepsy. But the oddest part was that no one in the local communities considered the individual victims abnormal, although it might appear like demonic possession of old.

The dance itself resembled an exorcism of the invisible spider within. In the church the victim lay down supine, groveling at first with fingers and nails extending toward the pavement like talons. Then she ran in circles, within a magic perimeter, before falling to the ground, where she beat the pavement rhythmically. She had turned into a spider dying! Jervis saw the psychic symbolism of the actions in the dance; De Martino, on the other hand, saw the external imposition of control and authority at every stage.

Historian J. F. C. Hecker, however, writing in 1832, saw tarantism as a latter-day Pugliese version of St Vitus's dance. This was an epidemic of wild dancing by groups of guilt-ridden survivors of the Black Death in the Rhine areas of Germany and Belgium, beginning with the events of 1374 in Aix-la-Chapelle. 'They formed circles hand in hand, and appearing to have lost all control over their senses, continued dancing, regardless of the by-standers, for hours together in wild delirium, until at length they fell to the ground in a state of exhaustion. Bystanders could control some of the fits by binding the victims tightly around the waist, while other accounts noted some success

with the use of tympany or other musical intervention. The clergy, however, were more concerned with the moral dangers the dancers presented, detailing ruinous disorders, the possibility of demonic possession, the excitation of 'secret desires' and opportunities for 'wild enjoyments'. Some priests attempted to exorcise victims, and to issue preventive regulations such as banning red cloth or the fashionable pointy-toed shoes. The phenomenon recalled the wandering bands of flagellants during the Black Death; Hecker was convinced that the epidemics of mania stemmed from the remembrance of sins and crimes committed during the plague.

Also called St Vitus's dance, the dancing mania is distinguishable from tarantism because it was a group phenomenon, and occurred sporadically in the late fourteenth and the fifteenth centuries in German lands. Its point of connection to tarantism, which peaked in the seventeenth century when St Vitus's dance had all but disappeared, was the musical cure or control. Hecker found no continuity of practice from medieval dancing mania to counter-Reformation tarantism.

But in both cases the power of saints was called on. There were several supernatural protectors related to dancing and disease. St Vitus was one of many Sicilian and southern Italian martyrs to the Emperor Diocletian's anti-Christian purges. The legend of his affiliation with the dancing mania of late medieval Europe dates from the fifteenth century.

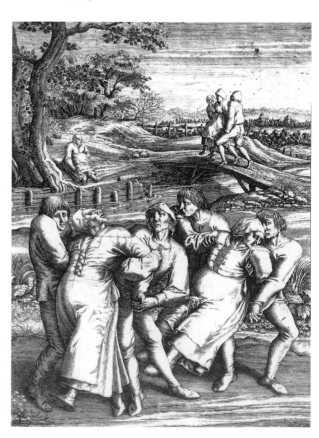

The St John festivals of midsummer date from a much earlier time; in the pagan calendar midsummer was celebrated with Bacchanalian festivities, involving dancing, and perhaps demonic possession and witchcraft. One view of the prehistory of tarantism would thus be that in this poor and illiterate region of Italy, Christianity had had but a meager toe-hold, and phenomena such as tarantism had to be explained and accommodated as best they could.

Angelo Turchini, the principal modern authority on tarantism, built on the work of De Martino and his colleagues, drawing together much of the historical arcana that would help to explain the antiquity and persistence of tarantism in Apulia. Following Hecker's lead, he looked for the saint. Vitus was not the saint for the *tarantati*. St Paul, however, had many associations with the disease. Two miracle-working relics are associated with him: 'St. Paul's Tongue', fossil shark's tooth, was used throughout this region of the Mediterranean as an amulet (so powerful that it could penetrate the rocks!); and St Paul's earth, from the cave where he stayed in M'dina, on the island of Malta. (By the seventeenth century St Paul's earth was

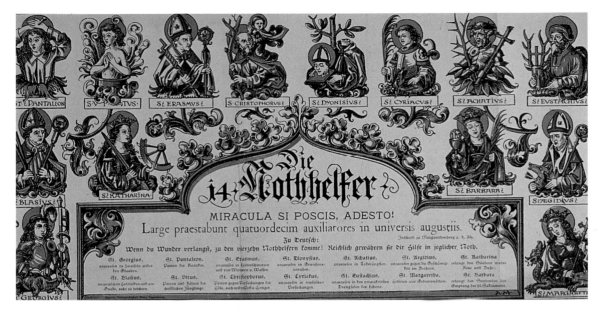

called *terra sigillata*, earth which had been stamped officially so that users could not be swindled.) It was held to be a powerful antidote to all kinds of animal and insect bites. St Paul was also said to have slept at a priest's house in Galatina, when fleeing his persecutors incognito. In gratitude to the religious man, St Paul blessed his well, rendering the water a ready remedy against all sorts of poisons: tarantulas, scorpions, vipers and so forth. And, as we have seen, it was to the church of San Paolo a Galatina, close to the well traditionally blessed by St Paul himself, that difficult cases of tarantism were brought in De Martino's day, and as recently as the 1970s.

The traditions attached to St Paul helped to give rise in the late Middle Ages to a group of wandering healers who styled themselves *sanpaolisti*, or healers of the house of St Paul; they charmed snakes and touted cure-alls for any variety of poison. Concern about the proliferation of such vagabond healers and soothsayers led to sixteenth-century studies into the nature and characteristics of antidotes; and it was not long after this that Epifanio Ferdinando wrote his classic description of tarantism, in 1621.

The story of tarantism is a beautiful illustration of the way in which the history of plagues and pestilences reveals the cultural associations and practices that define and control what disease is, when it is seen, when it is deemed a problem, why cures work, how diseases are born and disappear. Rite and ritual are never far away.

BIBLIOGRAPHY

Hecker, J. F. C. German 1st edn, 1832. 'The Dancing Mania of the Middle Ages' (trans. B. G. Babbington). Reprinted in *The Humboldt Library of Popular Science Literature*, vol. 7. New York.

Sigerist, Henry E. 1943, reprinted 1962. *Civilization and Disease*, Chapter 11. Chicago.

Turchini, Angelo. 1987. *Morso, morbo, morte: la tarantola fra cultura medica e terapia popolare*. Milan. (This work, the best single book on the topic, is unfortunately not available in English. I have relied on it for this chapter.)

Fourteen saints who provide help against specific troubles. St Vitus is second from the left on the top row.

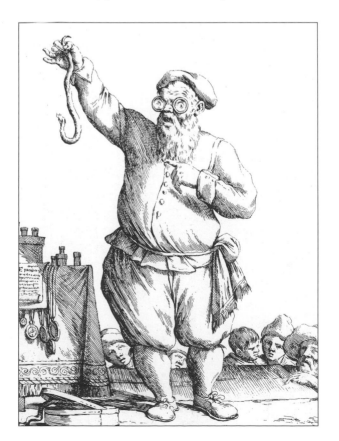

A seventeenth-century charlatan holding a charmed snake aloft. The proliferation of such 'curers' suggests that they may have carried antidotes to certain poisons among their charms.

GLOSSARY

amine – a derivative of ammonia. Casmir Funk who coined the word 'vitamin' believed this to be the missing vital element that produced susceptibilitiy to nutritional diseases. Hence vitaamine, or 'vitamine'. When it was later discovered that the amine hypothesis would not stand up the final 'e' was dropped.

arbovirus – the term comes from *ar*thropod – *bo*rne and virus. These are any group of viruses transmitted to humans by mosquitoes and ticks.

arteriole – a tiny arterial branch, especially one in close proximity to a capillary.

autoclave – a device that sterilizes with steam under pressure. It has a gauge that regulates the pressure and thus the heat.

bleb – a large flaccid bladderlike cell or cavity. In anatomical and pathological usage a bleb is filled with fluid.

bacillus - any of the rod-shaped bacteria of the genus Bacillus that require oxygen to live. They often occur in chainlike formations. See also under virus/bacterium.

bacterium – see under virus/bacterium.

clinical/subclinical – clinical pertains to direct observation and treatment of patients. A disease with clinical symptoms is one that is recognizable, as distinct from a subclinical illness without clinical manifestations, which can be a mild form of the illness or in an early stage.

commensal – means literally eating at the same table. In biological terms commensalism can imply a relationship between two organisms in which one benefits from, but does not harm the other. Mice benefiting from living close to humans is an example.

dermatitis – inflammation of the skin.

diathesis – a congential, frequently inherited susceptibility or predisposition to a disease or group of diseases, or to some sort of structural or metabolic disorder.

edema – a swelling caused by an excessive accumulation of serous fluid in the tissues.

endemic – see under epidemic, endemic, pandemic.

enzootic/epizootic – when a disease is present in an animal community at all times but causing only a limited number of cases it is said to be enzootic. When it attacks a large number of animals simultaneously in any region it is called epizootic.

epidemic, endemic, pandemic – when a disease suddenly appears to attack many people in the same region at roughly the same time it is called *epidemic*. When a disease is always present it is called *endemic*. And when an epidemic disease becomes widely distributed thoroughout a region, continent or the globe it is called *pandemic*.

etiology (also **aetiology**) – the cause, origin, or reason for a disease.

filtrate – to put through a filter.

flavivius – the yellow-fever virus.

foci – plural of focus. In this case the areas from which a disease radiates.

formications – a sensation of small insects crawling over the skin.

genera – plural of genus, a taxonomic category below a family and above a species. Can also mean simply a class or group with common attributes.

germ – a pathogenic microorganism.

heme/non-heme – a chemical distinction between the iron derived from animal sources (heme) and vegetable sources.

host – see under parasite/host.

inoculum – the substance used in inoculation.

microparasites – parasitic microorganisms.

miliary – can mean a disease marked by small skin lesions that look like millet seeds. In the case of miliary tuberculosis the meaning is an acute form of the disease characterized by very small tubercles in various body organs caused by their spread through the blood stream.

morbidity/mortality – a disease can be characterized by the morbidity (meaning sickness) and mortality (deaths) it produces in a population.

morbillivirus – the virus that causes measles.

morphology – the structure and form of an organism.

mycobacteria – plural for mycobacterium, a fast-acting microorganism that resembles the bacillus that causes tuberculosis. It is found in pulmonary infections and is the object of much ongoing research.

nanometer – one billionth of a meter.

neuron (also **neurone**) – a nerve-cell, actually any of the conducting cells of the nervous system.

nosological – pertaining to nosology, the classifaction of disease.

oncological – pertaining to oncology, the scientific study and treatment of tumors.

pandemic – see under epidemic, endemic, pandemic.

parasite/host – in the context of this book parasites mean pathogens (see below) that invade human hosts.

pathogen – any disease-producing microorganism.

pathology – the term meaning the study of the causes, processes, developments and consequences of disease. It can also mean the manifestations of disease.

penicillin – any of several antibiotic compounds obtained from penicillin molds or produced biosyhnthetically that are used to prevent and treat a variety of infections and diseases.

plasmodium – malarial parasites.

postprimary infection – a secondary infection following an initial infection, often after a considerable length of time.

prodromal – symptoms at the onset of a disease.

pure culture – a culture of a single species of cell that is free of contamination.

sepsis – the presence in the blood or other tissues of pathogenic organisms or their toxins. Infection.

serotype – the kind of microorganism as determined by the types and combinations of constituent antigens present in the cell.

serum – the clear fluid obtained when whole blood is separated into its solid and liquid components. Also the fluid from the tissues of immunized animals used as an antitoxin.

spirochete – a spiral bacterium and a general term for any microorganism of the order Spirochaetales one family of which causes the treponemal diseasesveneral and nonveneral syphilis, yaws, and pinta. See also under treponeme.

Streptococcus – any of the often pathogenic bacteria of the genus *Streptococcus* that generally occur in chains. The streptococci are responsible for numerous diseases among them scarlet fever, eryysipelas, puerperal sepsis and impetigo.

subclinical – see above under clinical.

sulfone – Sulfo is a prefix naming a set of chemical compounds indicating the presence of divalent sulphur. Sulfonamides were the wonder drugs that preceded anitbiotics. They affect bacterial metabolism and prevent their multiplication in the host.

sylvatic – sylvan; pertaining to the woods. In the case of plague it means spreading among creatures of the wild such as ground squirrels and other rodents. For enzootic see above.

treponeme – any of the spirochetes belonging to the genus *treponema* that cause syphilis and yaws among other diseases.

variolation – inoculation with the virus of smallpox as practiced before vaccination. Scabs from a smallpox victim might be scratched into the skin, or applied to the nasal membranes, or ingested.

vector – from *vehere* meaning to carry. A carrier which transports disease agents from one host to another such as the mosquitoes that sspread the protozoa of malaria or the virus of yellow fever.

vibrio – a microorganism of the genus Vibrio. Vibrio cholerae is the etiologic agent of Asiatic cholera.

virgin soil epidemic – a disease is said to have found 'virgin soil' when it erupts among a people never before exposed to it.

virus – one of a very large group of agents some of which cause infectious disease against which we vaccinate but for which we have yet to find a cure. Viruses range in severity from the common cold to influenza to AIDS. Accepted bacterial forms which together make up a large group of unicellular and multicellular organisms are larger than viruses. Many are important in the production of chemicals, enzymes, and antibiotics. Many others, however, have pathogenic properties that cause a wide range of disease in humans, animals, and plants. Examples include the bacillus, a bacterium that produces bacillary dysentery, bacillary pneumonia, or some bacteria of the *Streptococcus* genus that cause scarlet fever and other illnesses. The discovery of bacteria in the last quarter of the nineteenth century led to the 'germ theory of disease' and the field of bacteriology, of which virology is an important offshoot.

PICTURE ACKNOWLEDGEMENTS

A.K.G. London: Page 32, 40 (bottom), 44, 48, 50–51, 56, 57, 59, 60, 72, 111, 140, 144, 146, 150, 164

Barnaby's Picture Library/Fotomas Index: 23, 29, 55, 80, 105, 107, 144 (bottom)

Bridgeman Art Library: 11 Private Collection, 15 Private Collection, 28 Walker Art Gallery, Liverpool, 33 Dulwich Picture Gallery, London, 35 Giraudon, 37 (bottom) Johnny van Haeften Gallery, London, 39 Vatican Museum, 42 Cheltenham Art Gallery & Museums, Gloucestershire, 45 Private Collection, 46 (top), Giraudon, 47 Giraudon, 51 (top) Giraudon, 52 Johnny van Haeften Gallery, London, 61 (top) Master and Fellows, Magdalene College, Cambridge, 62 Peter Willi, 63 Musee des Beaux-Arts, Marseilles, 64 Guildhall Library, Corporation of London, 65 (top) Biblioteca National, Madrid, 66 York City Art Gallery, 68 **British Library**: 71 (top) University of Dundee, 71 (bottom) Library of Congress, Washington D.C, 74 (top) Lauros/Giraudon, 82 Munch-museet, Oslo, 83 Library of Congress, Washington D.C, 85 National Maritime Museum, London, 88 Private Collection, 90 O'Shea Gallery, London, 94 (top) O'Shea Gallery, London, 103 Prado, Madrid, 106 Private Collection, 113 The Trustees of the Weston Park Foundation, 115 (bottom) Bibliotheque Nationale, Paris, 117 Private Collection, 120 National Palace, Mexico City/Giraudon, 123 British Library, 126 Free Library, Philadelphia, 128 Private Collection, 132 Christopher Wood Gallery, London, 134 Private Collection, 136 Royal Holloway and Bedford New College, Surrey, 155 Glasgow University Library, 156 Bibliotheque Nationale, Paris, 157 (top) Barber's Hall, London, 158 Galerie de Jonckheere, Paris, 165 Giraudon.

Corbis-Bettmann: 9, 34 (bottom), 43, 49, 73, 86, 87, 91, 92, 95, 97, 101, 104–105, 115 (top), 118, 119, 120 (bottom), 121, 122, 129, 131, 135, 139, 142, 146 (top), 151, 152, 160, 162

E.T.Archive: 7, 11, 21, 22 (bottom), 25, 26, 27, 30, 31, 34 (top), 36 (bottom), 40 (top), 41 (top), 53 (bottom), 70 (bottom), 74, 77 (bottom), 79 (right), 84, 96, 99, 100, 102, 108, 109, 137

Mary Evans Picture Library: 19, 29, 38, 54, 61 (bottom), 62 (bottom), 69 (bottom), 75, 77 (top), 110, 112 (top), 138, 150, 153

John Farley: 22 (top)

Clark Spencer Larsen: 12, 13

Wellcome Institute Library, London: Cover, 10, 14, 16, 17, 18, 36 (top), 37 (top), 41(bottom), 46 (bottom), 53 (top), 65 (bottom), 67, 69 (top), 70 (top), 76, 78, 79 (left), 81, 89, 93, 94 (bottom), 98, 103 (bottom), 108 (bottom), 112 (bottom), 125, 126 (top), 127, 129 (bottom), 130, 133, 134, 141, 143, 147, 148, 149, 157 (bottom), 159, 161, 163, 166, 167, 168, 169

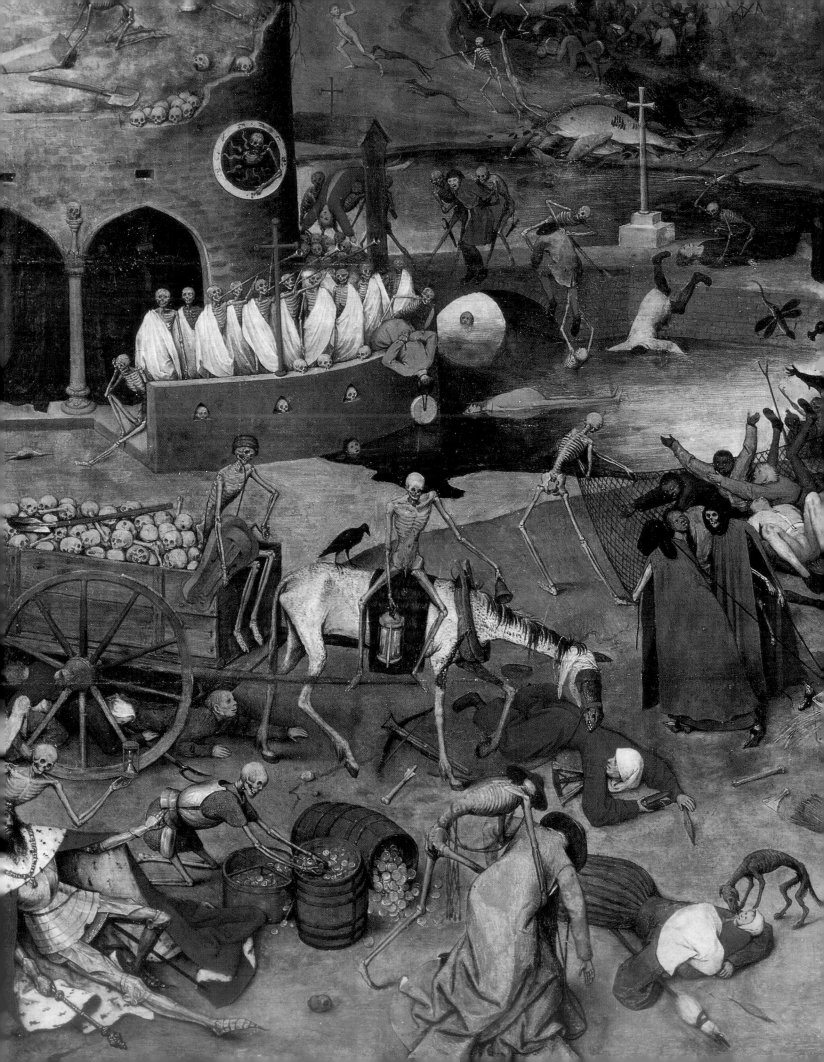